Management of severe malnutrition:
a manual for physicians and other senior health workers

Management of severe malnutrition:
a manual for physicians and other senior health workers

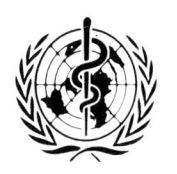

World Health Organization
Geneva
1999

WHO Library Cataloguing in Publication Data

Management of severe malnutrition: a manual for physicians and other senior health workers.

1.Child nutrition disorders – therapy   2.Nutrition disorders – therapy   3.Manuals   4.Guidelines

ISBN 92 4 154511 9 (NLM Classification: WD 101)

The World Health Organization welcomes requests for permission to reproduce or translate its publications, in part or in full. Applications and enquiries should be addressed to the Office of Publications, World Health Organization, Geneva, Switzerland, which will be glad to provide the latest information on any changes made to the text, plans for new editions, and reprints and translations already available.

© **World Health Organization 1999**

Publications of the World Health Organization enjoy copyright protection in accordance with the provisions of Protocol 2 of the Universal Copyright Convention. All rights reserved.

The designations employed and the presentation of the material in this publication do not imply the expression of any opinion whatsoever on the part of the Secretariat of the World Health Organization concerning the legal status of any country, territory, city or area or of its authorities, or concerning the delimitation of its frontiers or boundaries.

The mention of specific companies or of certain manufacturers' products does not imply that they are endorsed or recommended by the World Health Organization in preference to others of a similar nature that are not mentioned. Errors and omissions excepted, the names of proprietary products are distinguished by initial capital letters.

Typeset in Hong Kong
Printed in England
97/11527–Best-set/Clays–8500

Contents

Preface	v
Acknowledgements	vi
1. Introduction	**1**
2. Treatment facilities	**3**
3. Evaluation of the malnourished child	**4**
3.1 Assessment of nutritional status and criteria for admission	4
3.2 History and physical examination	5
3.3 Laboratory tests	5
4. Initial treatment	**7**
4.1 Principles of management	7
4.2 Hypoglycaemia	7
4.3 Hypothermia	8
4.4 Dehydration and septic shock	8
Diagnosis	8
Treatment of dehydration	9
Treatment of septic shock	12
4.5 Dietary treatment	12
Formula diets for severely malnourished children	13
Feeding on admission	13
Nasogastric feeding	14
Feeding after the appetite improves	15
Milk intolerance	16
Recording food intake	16
4.6 Infections	16
Bacterial infections	16
Measles and other viral infections	17
4.7 Vitamin deficiencies	17
Vitamin A deficiency	17
Other vitamin deficiencies	18
4.8 Very severe anaemia	18
4.9 Congestive heart failure	18
4.10 Dermatosis of kwashiorkor	19
5. Rehabilitation	**20**
5.1 Principles of management	20
5.2 Nutritional rehabilitation	20
Feeding children under 24 months	20
Feeding children over 24 months	21
Folic acid and iron	21
Assessing progress	22
5.3 Emotional and physical stimulation	22
The environment	23
Play activities	23
Physical activities	23

5.4	Teaching parents how to prevent malnutrition from recurring	24
5.5	Preparation for discharge	24
	Criteria for discharge	24
	Appropriate diets	24
	Immunization	25
	Planning follow-up	25

6. Follow-up — 26

7. Failure to respond to treatment — 27
- 7.1 General principles — 27
- 7.2 Problems with the treatment facility — 27
  - Type of facility — 27
  - Staff — 28
  - Inaccurate weighing machines — 28
  - Problems with preparing or giving food — 28
- 7.3 Problems with individual children — 29
  - Feeding — 29
  - Infection — 30
  - Serious underlying disease — 33
- 7.4 Learning from failure — 34

8. Management of malnutrition in disaster situations and refugee camps — 35
- 8.1 General considerations — 35
- 8.2 Establishing a therapeutic feeding centre — 35
  - Location and capacity — 35
  - Water supply and sanitation — 35
  - Cooking facilities and supplies — 35
  - Staff — 35
- 8.3 Criteria for enrolment and discharge — 35
- 8.4 Principles of management — 36
- 8.5 Evaluation of the therapeutic feeding centre — 36

9. Malnutrition in adolescents and adults — 37
- 9.1 Principles of management — 37
- 9.2 Classification of malnutrition — 37
  - Adults (over 18 years) — 37
  - Adolescents (10–18 years) — 38
- 9.3 History and physical examination — 38
- 9.4 Initial treatment — 38
- 9.5 Rehabilitation — 39
- 9.6 Criteria for discharge — 39
- 9.7 Failure to respond to treatment — 39

References — 40

Appendices — 41
1. NCHS/WHO normalized reference values for weight-for-height and weight-for-length — 41
2. Sample recording form — 43
3. Physiological basis for treatment of severe malnutrition — 50
4. Composition of mineral and vitamin mixes — 53
5. Desirable daily nutrient intake during initial phase of treatment — 54
6. Drug dosages for treatment of infections — 55
7. Toys for severely malnourished children — 58
8. Sample curriculum for play therapy — 59

Preface

Malnutrition remains one of the most common causes of morbidity and mortality among children throughout the world. Approximately 9% of children below 5 years of age suffer from wasting (weight-for-height below -2 standard deviations (<-2 SD) of the National Center for Health Statistics (NCHS)/WHO reference values) and are at risk of death or severe impairment of growth and psychological development.

This manual is based on *The treatment and management of severe protein–energy malnutrition*, which was published by WHO in 1981. Since then, many advances have been made in the treatment of severe malnutrition. An improved oral rehydration salts (ORS) solution has been developed for the treatment of dehydration. Advances in knowledge of the physiological roles of micronutrients have led to improved dietary management during the initial phase of treatment. It has been shown that physical and psychological stimulation, as well as care and affection, are necessary during the rehabilitation phase in order to prevent retardation of growth and psychological development.

This manual provides guidelines for the treatment of severely malnourished children (below 5 years of age) in hospitals and health centres. The treatment of severely malnourished adolescents and adults is also briefly considered. The manual is intended for health personnel working at central and district level, including physicians, nurses, midwives and auxiliaries.

Acknowledgements

The World Health Organization is particularly grateful to Dr M.H.N. Golden, University of Aberdeen, Aberdeen, Scotland, for his extensive contribution to the development of the final draft of this manual. It also thanks Professor J. Waterlow, London School of Hygiene and Tropical Medicine, London, England, for his assistance in the development of the initial draft. The World Health Organization also acknowledges the valuable contributions of the many experts who assisted in the development of the manual, including: Dr A. Ashworth, London School of Hygiene and Tropical Medicine, London, England; Dr M. Behar, Geneva, Switzerland; Ms R. Bhatia, Office of the United Nations High Commissioner for Refugees (UNHCR), Geneva, Switzerland; Dr M. Bolaert, *Médecins sans frontières*, Brussels, Belgium; Dr F. Chew, Institute of Nutrition of Central America and Panama (INCAP), Guatemala; Dr S. Grantham-McGregor, Institute of Child Health, London, England; Dr G. Lopez de Romana, Institute of Nutritional Studies, Lima, Peru; Dr V. Reddy, National Institute of Nutrition, Hyderabad, India; Dr B. Schürch, International Dietary Energy Consultancy Group (IDECG), Lausanne, Switzerland; Dr N. Scrimshaw, United Nations University, Boston, MA, USA; and Dr B. Torun, INCAP, Guatemala. It is also grateful to the staff of hospitals in Bangladesh, Brazil, India and Viet Nam and *Action contre la faim*, Paris, France, who provided many valuable practical comments on the final draft.

The following WHO staff members provided substantial technical contributions and comments: Dr K. Bailey, Programme of Nutrition, WHO, Geneva, Switzerland; Dr D. Benbouzid, Programme of Nutrition, WHO, Geneva, Switzerland; Dr G. Clugston, Programme of Nutrition, WHO, Geneva, Switzerland; Dr B. de Benoist, WHO Regional Office for Africa, Brazzaville, Congo; Dr M. de Onis, Programme of Nutrition, WHO, Geneva, Switzerland; Dr O. Fontaine, Division of Child Health and Development, WHO, Geneva, Switzerland; Dr S. Khanum, WHO Regional Office for South-East Asia, New Dehli, India; and Dr N.F. Pierce, Division of Child Health and Development, WHO, Geneva, Switzerland.

The financial support of IDECG and UNHCR towards the development and publication of this manual is also gratefully acknowledged.

1.
Introduction

This manual provides practical guidelines for the management of patients with severe malnutrition.[1] It seeks to promote the best available therapy so as to reduce the risk of death, shorten the length of time spent in hospital, and facilitate rehabilitation and full recovery. Emphasis is given here to the management of severely malnourished children; the management of severely malnourished adults and adolescents is also considered briefly.

Severe malnutrition is both a medical and a social disorder. That is, the medical problems of the child result, in part, from the social problems of the home in which the child lives. Malnutrition is the end result of chronic nutritional and, frequently, emotional deprivation by carers who, because of poor understanding, poverty or family problems, are unable to provide the child with the nutrition and care he or she requires. Successful management of the severely malnourished child requires that both medical and social problems be recognized and corrected. If the illness is viewed as being only a medical disorder, the child is likely to relapse when he or she returns home, and other children in the family will remain at risk of developing the same problem.

Table 1. Time-frame for the management of a child with severe malnutrition

Activity	Initial treatment:		Rehabilitation:	Follow-up:
	days 1–2	days 3–7	weeks 2–6	weeks 7–26
Treat or prevent: hypoglycaemia hypothermia dehydration	------→ ------→ ------→			
Correct electrolyte imbalance	---------------------------→			
Treat infection	------------→			
Correct micronutrient deficiencies	←— without iron —*—with iron—→			
Begin feeding	------------→			
Increase feeding to recover lost weight ("catch-up growth")			---------------------→	
Stimulate emotional and sensorial development		---------------------------------→		
Prepare for discharge			----------→	

[1] "Malnutrition" and "malnourished" are used as synonyms of "undernutrition" and "undernourished", respectively.

Management of the child with severe malnutrition is divided into three phases. These are:

- *Initial treatment:* life-threatening problems are identified and treated in a hospital or a residential care facility, specific deficiencies are corrected, metabolic abnormalities are reversed and feeding is begun.
- *Rehabilitation:* intensive feeding is given to recover most of the lost weight, emotional and physical stimulation are increased, the mother or carer is trained to continue care at home, and preparations are made for discharge of the child.
- *Follow-up:* after discharge, the child and the child's family are followed to prevent relapse and assure the continued physical, mental and emotional development of the child.

A typical time-frame for the management of a child with severe malnutrition is shown in Table 1.

Successful management of the severely malnourished child does not require sophisticated facilities and equipment or highly qualified personnel. It does, however, require that each child be treated with proper care and affection, and that each phase of treatment be carried out properly by appropriately trained and dedicated health workers. When this is done, the risk of death can be substantially reduced[1] and the opportunity for full recovery greatly improved.

---

[1] For the purposes of this manual, a case-fatality rate of >20% is considered unacceptable, 11–20% is poor, 5–10% is moderate, 1–4% is good and <1% is excellent.

2.
Treatment facilities

Residential care is essential for initial treatment and for the beginning of rehabilitation of a child with severe malnutrition. The child should be admitted to hospital, preferably to a special nutrition unit, which is an area in a general hospital that is dedicated to the initial management and rehabilitation of severe malnutrition. When the child has completed the initial phase of treatment, has no complications, and is eating satisfactorily and gaining weight (usually 2–3 weeks after admission), he or she can usually be managed at a non-residential nutrition rehabilitation centre. A nutrition rehabilitation centre is a day hospital, primary health centre or similar facility that provides daytime care by staff trained in the rehabilitation of malnourished children. The child sleeps at home, is brought to the centre each morning, and returns home each evening. Close cooperation between the hospital and centre is necessary to ensure continuity of care for the child and facilitate returning the child quickly to hospital, should a serious problem develop. In urban areas, nutrition rehabilitation centres should preferably be established close to hospital facilities. In areas where there are no specialized centres, the hospital must continue to provide care until the child is ready for discharge. Important features of residential and non-residential treatment facilities are compared in Table 2.

*Table 2. **Comparison of residential and non-residential facilities for treating severely malnourished children***

Feature	Residential care (hospital)	Non-residential care (nutrition rehabilitation centre)
Daily transport required	No	Yes
Number and level of training of staff	Large number, formally trained	Fewer staff, informally trained
Diagnostic, consultant and support services	Usually available	Patient must be taken to hospital
Emergency care	Available at all times	Patient may need to be taken to hospital
Care available 24 h per day	Yes	No
Patient can be fed throughout the night	Yes	No
Inappropriate remedies can be given at home	No	Yes
Child separated from mother	Sometimes	No
Rate of staff turnover	High	Low
Risk of cross-infection	High	Moderate
Intimidating for parents and children	Often	Sometimes
Financial cost	High	Moderate
Cost in terms of parental time required	Moderate	High

3. Evaluation of the malnourished child

When first seen, the child must be examined, a history taken and a decision made on the treatment to be given. Treatment should be started as soon as these tasks have been completed; details of the history and examination should be recorded later. Very sick children respond badly to frequent handling; they should not be taken for X-rays initially and should remain in bed while clinical specimens are taken.

3.1 Assessment of nutritional status and criteria for admission

The assessment of nutritional status according to weight-for-height (or length),[1] height (or length)-for-age[1] and oedema is summarized in Table 3. Also shown are the criteria for classifying severe malnutrition as "oedematous", "severely wasted" or "severely stunted". Reference values for weight-for-height or length are given in Appendix 1.

Children whose weight-for-height is below −3 SD or less than 70% of the median NCHS/WHO reference values (termed "severely wasted"), or who have symmetrical oedema involving at least the feet (termed "oedematous malnutrition") are severely malnourished. They should be admitted to hospital where they can be observed, treated and fed day and night.

Table 3. Classification of malnutrition[a]

	Classification	
	Moderate malnutrition	Severe malnutrition (type)[b]
Symmetrical oedema	No	Yes (oedematous malnutrition)[c]
Weight-for-height	−3 ≤ SD-score <−2[d] (70–79%)[e]	SD-score <−3 (<70%) (severe wasting)[f]
Height-for-age	−3 ≤ SD-score <−2 (85–89%)	SD-score <−3 (<85%) (severe stunting)

[a] For further information about anthropometric indicators, see reference 1.
[b] The diagnoses are not mutually exclusive.
[c] This includes kwashiorkor and marasmic kwashiorkor in older classifications. However, to avoid confusion with the clinical syndrome of kwashiorkor, which includes other features, the term "oedematous malnutrition" is preferred.
[d] Below the median NCHS/WHO reference; the SD-score is defined as the deviation of the value for an individual from the median value of the reference population, divided by the standard deviation of the reference population.

$$\text{SD-score} = \frac{(\text{observed value}) - (\text{median reference value})}{\text{standard deviation of reference population}}$$

[e] Percentage of the median NCHS/WHO reference (see footnote in Appendix 1).
[f] This corresponds to marasmus (without oedema) in the Wellcome clinical classification (2, 3), and to grade III malnutrition in the Gomez system (4). However, to avoid confusion, the term "severe wasting" is preferred.

---

[1] In this manual length and height, as well as weight-for-length and weight-for-height, are used interchangeably. Children who are below 24 months, less than 85 cm tall, or too ill to stand should have their *length* measured while they are lying down. Children who are 24 months or more and 85 cm or more tall, and who are able to stand should have their *height* measured.

3. Evaluation of the malnourished child

Stunted children are usually considered to have a milder, chronic form of malnutrition. Their condition can rapidly worsen, however, with the onset of complications such as diarrhoea, respiratory infections or measles. Stunted children may be satisfactorily managed in the community, rather than in hospital. Management of children with severe stunting should follow guidelines for "preparation for discharge" (see section 5.5).

3.2 History and physical examination

A checklist for taking the child's medical history and conducting the physical examination is given in the box below. It helps to use a printed proforma so that the information is collected and recorded in a standard manner. A sample recording form is given in Appendix 2, which may be adapted to local conditions.

Checklist of points for taking the child's medical history and conducting the physical examination

Medical history:
- Usual diet before current episode of illness
- Breastfeeding history
- Food and fluids taken in past few days
- Recent sinking of eyes
- Duration and frequency of vomiting or diarrhoea, appearance of vomit or diarrhoeal stools
- Time when urine was last passed
- Contact with people with measles or tuberculosis
- Any deaths of siblings
- Birth weight
- Milestones reached (sitting up, standing, etc.)
- Immunizations

Physical examination:
- Weight and length or height
- Oedema
- Enlargement or tenderness of liver, jaundice
- Abdominal distension, bowel sounds, "abdominal splash" (a splashing sound in the abdomen)
- Severe pallor
- Signs of circulatory collapse: cold hands and feet, weak radial pulse, diminished consciousness
- Temperature: hypothermia or fever
- Thirst
- Eyes: corneal lesions indicative of vitamin A deficiency
- Ears, mouth, throat: evidence of infection
- Skin: evidence of infection or purpura
- Respiratory rate and type of respiration: signs of pneumonia or heart failure
- Appearance of faeces

3.3 Laboratory tests

Where facilities permit, the tests given in Table 4 may help to diagnose specific problems. They are not needed, however, to guide or monitor treatment. The interpretation of test results is frequently altered by malnutrition. For this reason, laboratory tests may misguide inexperienced workers. The most important guide to treatment is frequent careful assessment of the child.

Table 4. Laboratory tests

Test	Result and significance
Tests that may be useful	
Blood glucose	Glucose concentration <54 mg/dl (3 mmol/l) is indicative of hypoglycaemia
Examination of blood smear by microscopy	Presence of malaria parasites is indicative of infection
Haemoglobin or packed-cell volume	Haemoglobin <40 g/l or packed-cell volume <12% is indicative of very severe anaemia
Examination and culture of urine specimen	Presence of bacteria on microscopy (or >10 leukocytes per high-power field) is indicative of infection
Examination of faeces by microscopy	Presence of blood is indicative of dysentery Presence of *Giardia* cysts or trophozoites is indicative of infection
Chest X-ray	Pneumonia causes less shadowing of the lungs in malnourished children than in well-nourished children Vascular engorgement is indicative of heart failure Bones may show rickets or fractures of the ribs
Skin test for tuberculosis	Often negative in children with tuberculosis or those previously vaccinated with BCG vaccine
Tests that are of little or no value	
Serum proteins	Not useful in management, but may guide prognosis
Test for human immunodeficiency virus (HIV)	Should not be done routinely; if done, should be accompanied by counselling of the child's parents and result should be confidential
Electrolytes	Rarely helpful and may lead to inappropriate therapy

4. Initial treatment

4.1 Principles of management

Children with severe malnutrition are often seriously ill when they first present for treatment. Wasting, anorexia and infections are common. Wherever possible, severely malnourished children should be referred to hospital. Successful initial management requires frequent, careful clinical evaluation and anticipation of common problems so they can be prevented, or recognized and treated at an early stage. The physiology of malnourished children is seriously abnormal; how this affects their management is summarized in Appendix 3.

Recently admitted children should be kept in a special area where they can be *constantly monitored*. Because they are very susceptible to infection, they should, if possible, be isolated from other patients. The child should not be kept near a window or in a draught, and windows should be closed at night. The child should be properly covered with clothes, including a hat, and blankets. Washing should be kept to a minimum and, if necessary, done during the day. When the child is washed he or she must be dried immediately and properly. The room temperature should be kept at 25–30 °C (77–86 °F). This will seem uncomfortably warm for active, fully clothed staff, but is necessary for small, immobile children who easily become hypothermic.

Intravenous infusions should be avoided except when essential, as for severe dehydration or septic shock. Intramuscular injections should be given with care in the buttock, using the smallest possible gauge needle and volume of fluid.

Initial treatment begins with admission to hospital and lasts until the child's condition is stable and his or her appetite has returned, which is usually after 2–7 days. If the initial phase takes longer than 10 days, the child is failing to respond and additional measures are required (see section 7). The principal tasks during initial treatment are:

— to treat or prevent hypoglycaemia and hypothermia;
— to treat or prevent dehydration and restore electrolyte balance;
— to treat incipient or developed septic shock, if present;
— to start to feed the child;
— to treat infection;
— to identify and treat any other problems, including vitamin deficiency, severe anaemia and heart failure.

These tasks are described in detail below.

4.2 Hypoglycaemia

All severely malnourished children are at risk of developing hypoglycaemia (blood glucose <54 mg/dl or <3 mmol/l), which is an important cause of death during the first 2 days of treatment. Hypoglycaemia may be caused by a serious systemic infection or can occur when a malnourished child has not been fed for 4–6 hours, as often happens during travel to hospital. To prevent hypoglycaemia the child should be fed at least every 2 or 3 hours day and night (see section 4.5).

Signs of hypoglycaemia include low body temperature (<36.5 °C), lethargy, limpness and loss of consciousness. Sweating and pallor do not usually occur in malnourished children with hypoglycaemia. Often, the only sign before death is drowsiness.

If hypoglycaemia is suspected, treatment should be given *immediately without laboratory confirmation*; it can do no harm, even if the diagnosis is incorrect. If the patient is conscious or can be roused and is able to drink, give 50 ml of 10% glucose or sucrose, or give F-75 diet by mouth (see section 4.5), whichever is available most quickly. If only 50% glucose solution is available, dilute one part to four parts of sterile water. Stay with the child until he or she is fully alert.

If the child is losing consciousness, cannot be aroused or has convulsions, give 5 ml/kg of body weight of sterile 10% glucose intravenously (IV), followed by 50 ml of 10% glucose or sucrose by nasogastric (NG) tube. If IV glucose cannot be given immediately, give the NG dose first. When the child regains consciousness, immediately begin giving F-75 diet or glucose in water (60 g/l). Continue frequent oral or NG feeding with F-75 diet to prevent a recurrence.

All malnourished children with suspected hypoglycaemia should also be treated with broad-spectrum antimicrobials for serious systemic infection (see section 4.6).

4.3 Hypothermia

Infants under 12 months, and those with marasmus, large areas of damaged skin or serious infections are highly susceptible to hypothermia. If the rectal temperature is below 35.5 °C (95.9 °F) or the underarm temperature is below 35.0 °C (95.0 °F), the child should be warmed. Either use the "kangaroo technique" by placing the child on the mother's bare chest or abdomen (skin-to-skin) and covering both of them, or clothe the child well (including the head), cover with a warmed blanket and place an incandescent lamp over, but not touching, the child's body. Fluorescent lamps are of no use and hot-water bottles are dangerous.

The rectal temperature must be measured every 30 minutes during rewarming with a lamp, as the child may rapidly become hyperthermic. The underarm temperature is not a reliable guide to body temperature during rewarming.

All hypothermic children must also be treated for hypoglycaemia (see section 4.2) and for serious systemic infection (see section 4.6).

4.4 Dehydration and septic shock

Dehydration and septic shock are difficult to differentiate in a child with severe malnutrition. Signs of hypovolaemia are seen in both conditions, and progressively worsen if treatment is not given. Dehydration progresses from "some" to "severe", reflecting 5–10% and >10% weight loss, respectively, whereas septic shock progresses from "incipient" to "developed", as blood flow to the vital organs decreases. Moreover, in many cases of septic shock there is a history of diarrhoea and some degree of dehydration, giving a mixed clinical picture.

Diagnosis

Many of the signs that are normally used to assess dehydration are unreliable in a child with severe malnutrition, making it difficult or impossible to detect dehydration reliably or determine its severity. Moreover, many signs of dehydration are also seen in septic shock. This has two results:

— dehydration tends to be overdiagnosed and its severity overestimated; and
— it is often necessary to treat the child for both dehydration and septic shock.

4. Initial treatment

(a) Signs of dehydration and/or septic shock that are reliable in a child with severe malnutrition include:

History of diarrhoea. A child with dehydration should have a history of watery diarrhoea. Small mucoid stools are commonly seen in severe malnutrition, but do not cause dehydration. A child with signs of dehydration, but without watery diarrhoea, should be treated as having septic shock.

Thirst. Drinking eagerly is a reliable sign of "some" dehydration. In infants this may be expressed as restlessness. Thirst is *not* a symptom of septic shock.

Hypothermia. When present, this is a sign of serious infection, including septic shock. It is *not* a sign of dehydration.

Sunken eyes. These are a helpful sign of dehydration, but only when the mother says the sunken appearance is recent.

Weak or absent radial pulse. This is a sign of shock, from either severe dehydration or sepsis. As hypovolaemia develops, the pulse rate increases and the pulse becomes weaker. If the pulse in the carotid, femoral or brachial artery is weak, the child is at risk of dying and must be treated urgently.

Cold hands and feet. This is a sign of both severe dehydration and septic shock. It should be assessed with the back of the hand.

Urine flow. Urine flow diminishes as dehydration or septic shock worsens. In severe dehydration or fully developed septic shock, no urine is formed.

(b) Signs of dehydration that are *not reliable* include:

Mental state. A severely malnourished child is usually apathetic when left alone and irritable when handled. As dehydration worsens, the child progressively loses consciousness. Hypoglycaemia, hypothermia and septic shock also cause reduced consciousness.

Mouth, tongue and tears. The salivary and lacrimal glands are atrophied in severe malnutrition, so the child usually has a dry mouth and absent tears. Breathing through the mouth also makes the mouth dry.

Skin elasticity. The loss of supporting tissues and absence of subcutaneous fat make the skin thin and loose. It flattens very slowly when pinched, or may not flatten at all. Oedema, if present, may mask diminished elasticity of the skin.

The clinical features of dehydration and septic shock are compared in Table 5.

(c) Additional signs of septic shock:

Incipient septic shock. The child is usually limp, apathetic and profoundly anorexic, but is neither thirsty nor restless.

Developed septic shock. The superficial veins, such as the external jugular and scalp veins, are dilated rather than constricted. The veins in the lungs may also become engorged, making the lungs stiffer than normal. For this reason the child may groan, grunt, have a shallow cough and appear to have difficulty breathing. As shock worsens, kidney, liver, intestinal or cardiac failure may occur. There may be vomiting of blood mixed with stomach contents ("coffee-ground vomit"), blood in the stool, and abdominal distension with "abdominal splash"; intestinal fluid may be visible on X-ray. When a child reaches this stage, survival is unlikely.

Treatment of dehydration

Whenever possible, a dehydrated child with severe malnutrition should be rehydrated

*Table 5. Comparison of clinical signs of **dehydration** and **septic shock** in the severely malnourished child*

Clinical sign	Some dehydration	Severe dehydration	Incipient septic shock	Developed septic shock
Watery diarrhoea	Yes	Yes	Yes or no[a]	Yes or no[a]
Thirst	Drinks eagerly[b]	Drinks poorly	No[a]	No[a]
Hypothermia	No	No	Yes[a] or no	Yes[a] or no
Sunken eyes	Yes[b,c]	Yes[b,c]	No[a]	No[a]
Weak or absent radial pulse	No[b]	Yes	Yes	Yes
Cold hands and feet	No[b]	Yes	Yes	Yes
Urine flow	Yes	No	Yes	No
Mental state	Restless, irritable[b]	Lethargic, comatose	Apathetic[a]	Lethargic
Hypoglycaemia	Sometimes	Sometimes	Sometimes	Sometimes

[a] Signs that may be useful in diagnosing septic shock.
[b] Signs that may be useful in diagnosing dehydration.
[c] If confirmed as recent by the mother.

orally. IV infusion easily causes overhydration and heart failure and should be used *only* when there are definite signs of shock.

Oral rehydration salts (ORS) solution for severely malnourished children

Because severely malnourished children are deficient in potassium and have abnormally high levels of sodium, the oral rehydration salts (ORS) solution should contain less sodium and more potassium than the standard WHO-recommended solution. Magnesium, zinc and copper should also be given to correct deficiencies of these minerals. The composition of the recommended ORS solution for severely malnourished children (ReSoMal) is given in Table 6.

ReSoMal is available commercially. However, ReSoMal can also be made by diluting one packet of the standard WHO-recommended ORS in 2 litres of water, instead of 1 litre, and adding 50 g of sucrose (25 g/l) and 40 ml (20 ml/l) of mineral mix solution[1] (see Appendix 4).

Amount of ReSoMal to give

Between 70 and 100 ml of ReSoMal per kg of body weight is usually enough to restore normal hydration. Give this amount over 12 hours, starting with 5 ml/kg every 30 minutes for the first 2 hours orally or by NG tube, and then 5–10 ml/kg per hour. This rate is slower than for children who are not severely malnourished. Reassess the child *at least* every hour. The exact amount to give should be determined by how much the child will drink, the amount of ongoing losses in the stool, and whether the child is vomiting and has any signs of overhydration, especially signs of heart failure. ReSoMal should be stopped if:

— the respiratory and pulse rates increase;
— the jugular veins become engorged; or
— there is increasing oedema (e.g. puffy eyelids).

Rehydration is completed when the child is no longer thirsty, urine is passed and any other signs of dehydration have disappeared. Fluids given to maintain hydration should

---

[1] Contains the mineral salts needed to prepare ReSoMal from the standard WHO-recommended ORS solution. The same salts are also added to the child's food (see section 4.5 and Appendix 4).

4. Initial treatment

Table 6. Composition of oral rehydration salts solution for severely malnourished children (ReSoMal)

Component	Concentration (mmol/l)
Glucose	125
Sodium	45
Potassium	40
Chloride	70
Citrate	7
Magnesium	3
Zinc	0.3
Copper	0.045
Osmolarity	300

be based on the child's willingness to drink and, if possible, the amount of ongoing losses in the stool. As a guide, children under 2 years should be given 50–100 ml (between one-quarter and one-half of a large cup) of ReSoMal after each loose stool, while older children should receive 100–200 ml. Continue this treatment until diarrhoea stops.

How to give ReSoMal

Children who can drink may be given the required amount as sips or by spoon every few minutes. However, malnourished children are weak and quickly become exhausted, so they may not continue to take enough fluid voluntarily. If this occurs, the solution should be given by NG tube at the same rate. An NG tube should be used in all weak or exhausted children, and in those who vomit, have fast breathing[1] or painful stomatitis.

Intravenous rehydration

The only indication for IV infusion in a severely malnourished child is circulatory collapse caused by severe dehydration or septic shock. Use one of the following solutions (in order of preference):

— half-strength Darrow's solution with 5% glucose (dextrose)
— Ringer's lactate solution with 5% glucose[2]
— 0.45% (half-normal) saline with 5% glucose.[2]

Give 15 ml/kg IV over 1 hour and monitor the child carefully for signs of overhydration. While the IV drip is being set up, also insert an NG tube and give ReSoMal through the tube (10 ml/kg per hour). Reassess the child after 1 hour. If the child is severely dehydrated, there should be an improvement with IV treatment and his or her respiratory and pulse rates should fall. In this case, repeat the IV treatment (15 mg/kg over 1 hour) and then switch to ReSoMal orally or by NG tube (10 ml/kg per hour) for up to 10 hours. If the child fails to improve after the first IV treatment and his or her radial pulse is still absent, then assume that the child has septic shock and treat accordingly (see page 12).

Feeding during rehydration

Breastfeeding should not be interrupted during rehydration. Begin to give the F-75 diet as soon as possible, orally or by NG tube, usually within 2–3 hours after starting

---

[1] Fast breathing is defined here as 50 breaths per minute or more if the child is aged 2 months up to 12 months and 40 breaths per minute or more if the child is aged 12 months up to 5 years.
[2] If possible, add sterile potassium chloride, 20 mmol/l.

rehydration (see section 4.5). If the child is alert and drinking, give the F-75 diet immediately, even before rehydration is completed. Usually the diet and ReSoMal are given in alternate hours. If the child vomits, give the diet by NG tube. When the child stops passing watery stools, continue feeding, as described in section 4.5.

Treatment of septic shock

All severely malnourished children with signs of incipient or developed septic shock should be treated for septic shock. This includes especially children with:

— signs of dehydration, but without a history of watery diarrhoea;
— hypothermia or hypoglycaemia;
— oedema and signs of dehydration.

Every child with septic shock should *immediately* be given broad-spectrum antibiotics (see section 4.6) and be kept warm to prevent or treat hypothermia (see section 4.3). The child should not be handled any more than is essential for treatment. Nor should the child be washed or bathed; after the child has defecated, his or her bottom can be cleaned with a damp cloth. Iron supplements should *not* be given. Other treatment is described below.

Incipient septic shock

The child should be fed promptly to prevent hypoglycaemia, using the F-75 diet with added mineral mix. As these children are nearly always anorexic, the diet must be given by NG tube. The amounts to be given and frequency of feeding are described in section 4.5.

Developed septic shock

Begin IV rehydration immediately, using one of the fluids listed on page 11. Give 15 ml/kg per hour. Observe the child carefully (every 5–10 minutes) for signs of overhydration and congestive heart failure (see section 4.9). As soon as the radial pulse becomes strong and the child regains consciousness, continue rehydration orally or by NG tube as described on pages 10–11. If signs of congestive heart failure develop or the child does not improve after 1 hour of IV therapy, give a blood transfusion (10 ml/kg slowly over at least 3 hours). If blood is not available, give plasma. If there are signs of liver failure (e.g. purpura, jaundice, enlarged tender liver), give a single dose of 1 mg of vitamin K_1 intramuscularly.

During the blood transfusion, nothing else should be given, so as to minimize the risk of congestive heart failure. If there is any sign of congestive heart failure (e.g. distension of the jugular veins, increasing respiratory rate or respiratory distress), give a diuretic (see section 4.9) and slow the rate of transfusion. Steroids, epinephrine or nikethamide are of no value and should *never* be used.

After the transfusion, begin to give F-75 diet by NG tube (see section 4.5). If the child develops increasing abdominal distension or vomits repeatedly, give the diet more slowly. If the problem does not resolve, stop feeding the child and give one of the fluids listed on page 11 by IV infusion at a rate of 2–4 ml/kg per hour. Also give 2 ml of 50% magnesium sulfate solution intramuscularly (IM).

4.5 Dietary treatment

Children who do not require other emergency treatment, especially for hypothermia, dehydration or septic shock, should immediately be given a formula diet. They should also continue to be breastfed.

4. Initial treatment

Formula diets for severely malnourished children

Almost all severely malnourished children have infections, impaired liver and intestinal function, and problems related to imbalance of electrolytes when first admitted to hospital. Because of these problems, they are unable to tolerate the usual amounts of dietary protein, fat and sodium. It is important, therefore, to begin feeding these children with a diet that is low in these nutrients, and high in carbohydrate. The daily nutrient requirements of severely malnourished children are given in Appendix 5.

Two formula diets, F-75 and F-100, are used for severely malnourished children. F-75 (75 kcal$_{th}$ or 315 kJ/100 ml), is used during the initial phase of treatment, while F-100 (100 kcal$_{th}$ or 420 kJ/100 ml) is used during the rehabilitation phase, after the appetite has returned. These formulas can easily be prepared from the basic ingredients: dried skimmed milk, sugar, cereal flour, oil, mineral mix and vitamin mix (see Table 7). They are also commercially available as powder formulations that are mixed with water.

The mineral mix supplies potassium, magnesium and other essential minerals (see Table 8); it *must* be added to the diet. The potassium deficit, present in all malnourished children, adversely affects cardiac function and gastric emptying. Magnesium is essential for potassium to enter cells and be retained. The mineral mix does not contain iron as this is withheld during the initial phase.

Table 7. Preparation of F-75 and F-100 diets

Ingredient	Amount	
	F-75[a–d]	F-100[e,f]
Dried skimmed milk	25 g	80 g
Sugar	70 g	50 g
Cereal flour	35 g	—
Vegetable oil	27 g	60 g
Mineral mix[g]	20 ml	20 ml
Vitamin mix[g]	140 mg	140 mg
Water to make	1000 ml	1000 ml

[a] To prepare the F-75 diet, add the dried skimmed milk, sugar, cereal flour and oil to some water and mix. Boil for 5–7 minutes. Allow to cool, then add the mineral mix and vitamin mix and mix again. Make up the volume to 1000 ml with water.

[b] A comparable formula can be made from 35 g of whole dried milk, 70 g of sugar, 35 g of cereal flour, 17 g of oil, 20 ml of mineral mix, 140 mg of vitamin mix and water to make 1000 ml. Alternatively, use 300 ml of fresh cows' milk, 70 g of sugar, 35 g of cereal flour, 17 g of oil, 20 ml of mineral mix, 140 mg of vitamin mix and water to make 1000 ml.

[c] Isotonic versions of F-75 (280 mOsmol/l), which contain maltodextrins instead of cereal flour and some of the sugar and which include all the necessary micronutrients, are available commercially.

[d] If cereal flour is not available or there are no cooking facilities, a comparable formula can be made from 25 g of dried skimmed milk, 100 g of sugar, 27 g of oil, 20 ml of mineral mix, 140 mg of vitamin mix and water to make 1000 ml. However, this formula has a high osmolarity (415 mOsmol/l) and may not be well tolerated by all children, especially those with diarrhoea.

[e] To prepare the F-100 diet, add the dried skimmed milk, sugar and oil to some warm boiled water and mix. Add the mineral mix and vitamin mix and mix again. Make up the volume to 1000 ml with water.

[f] A comparable formula can be made from 110 g of whole dried milk, 50 g of sugar, 30 g of oil, 20 ml of mineral mix, 140 mg of vitamin mix and water to make 1000 ml. Alternatively, use 880 ml of fresh cows' milk, 75 g of sugar, 20 g of oil, 20 ml of mineral mix, 140 mg of vitamin mix and water to make 1000 ml.

[g] See Appendix 4. If only small amounts of feed are being prepared, it will not be feasible to prepare the vitamin mix because of the small amounts involved. In this case, give a proprietary multivitamin supplement. Alternatively, a combined mineral and vitamin mix for malnourished children is available commercially and can be used in the above diets.

Feeding on admission

To avoid overloading the intestine, liver and kidneys, it is essential that food be given frequently and in small amounts. Children who are unwilling to eat should be fed by NG

Table 8. Composition of F-75 and F-100 diets

Constituent	Amount per 100 ml	
	F-75	F-100
Energy	75 kcal$_{th}$ (315 kJ)	100 kcal$_{th}$ (420 kJ)
Protein	0.9 g	2.9 g
Lactose	1.3 g	4.2 g
Potassium	3.6 mmol	5.9 mmol
Sodium	0.6 mmol	1.9 mmol
Magnesium	0.43 mmol	0.73 mmol
Zinc	2.0 mg	2.3 mg
Copper	0.25 mg	0.25 mg
Percentage of energy from:		
protein	5%	12%
fat	32%	53%
Osmolarity	333 mOsmol/l	419 mOsmol/l

tube (do *not* use IV feeding). Children who can eat should be given the diet every 2, 3 or 4 hours, day and night. If vomiting occurs, both the amount given at each feed and the interval between feeds should be reduced.

The F-75 diet should be given to all children during the initial phase of treatment. The child should be given at least 80 kcal$_{th}$ or 336 kJ/kg, but no more than 100 kcal$_{th}$ or 420 kJ/kg per day. If less than 80 kcal$_{th}$ or 336 kJ/kg per day are given, the tissues will continue to be broken down and the child will deteriorate. If more than 100 kcal$_{th}$ or 420 kJ/kg per day are given, the child may develop a serious metabolic imbalance.

Table 9 shows the amount of diet needed at each feed to achieve an intake of 100 kcal$_{th}$ or 420 kJ/kg per day. For example, if a child weighing 7.0 kg is given the F-75 diet every 2 hours, each feed should be 75 ml. During the initial phase of treatment, maintain the volume of F-75 feed at 130 ml/kg per day, but gradually decrease the frequency of feeding and increase the volume of each feed until you are giving the child feeds 4-hourly (6 feeds per day).

Nearly all malnourished children have poor appetites when first admitted to hospital. Patience and coaxing are needed to encourage the child to complete each feed. The child should be fed from a cup and spoon; feeding bottles should *never* be used, even for very young infants, as they are an important source of infection. Children who are very weak may be fed using a dropper or a syringe. While being fed, the child should always be held securely in a sitting position on the attendant's or mother's lap. Children should never be left alone in bed to feed themselves.

Nasogastric feeding

Despite coaxing and patience, many children will not take sufficient diet by mouth during the first few days of treatment. Common reasons include a very poor appetite, weakness and painful stomatitis. Such children should be fed using a NG tube. However, NG feeding should end as soon as possible. At each feed, the child should first be offered the diet orally. After the child has taken as much as he or she wants, the remainder should be given by NG tube. The NG tube should be removed when the child is taking three-quarters of the day's diet orally, or takes two consecutive feeds fully by mouth. If over the next 24 hours the child fails to take 80 kcal$_{th}$ or 336 kJ/kg, the tube should be reinserted. If the child develops abdominal distension during NG feeding, give 2 ml of a 50% solution of magnesium sulfate IM.

The NG tube should always be aspirated before fluids are administered. It should also be properly fixed so that it cannot move to the lungs during feeding. NG feeding should be done by experienced staff.

4. Initial treatment

Table 9. Determining the amount of diet to give at each feed to achieve a daily intake of 100 kcal$_{th}$ or 420 kJ/kg

Weight of child (kg)	Volume of F-75 per feed (ml)[a]		
	Every 2 hours (12 feeds)	Every 3 hours (8 feeds)	Every 4 hours (6 feeds)
2.0	20	30	45
2.2	25	35	50
2.4	25	40	55
2.6	30	45	55
2.8	30	45	60
3.0	35	50	65
3.2	35	55	70
3.4	35	55	75
3.6	40	60	80
3.8	40	60	85
4.0	45	65	90
4.2	45	70	90
4.4	50	70	95
4.6	50	75	100
4.8	55	80	105
5.0	55	80	110
5.2	55	85	115
5.4	60	90	120
5.6	60	90	125
5.8	65	95	130
6.0	65	100	130
6.2	70	100	135
6.4	70	105	140
6.6	75	110	145
6.8	75	110	150
7.0	75	115	155
7.2	80	120	160
7.4	80	120	160
7.6	85	125	165
7.8	85	130	170
8.0	90	130	175
8.2	90	135	180
8.4	90	140	185
8.6	95	140	190
8.8	95	145	195
9.0	100	145	200
9.2	100	150	200
9.4	105	155	205
9.6	105	155	210
9.8	110	160	215
10.0	110	160	220

[a] Rounded to the nearest 5 ml.

Feeding after the appetite improves

If the child's appetite improves, treatment has been successful. The initial phase of treatment ends when the child becomes hungry. This indicates that infections are coming under control, the liver is able to metabolize the diet, and other metabolic abnormalities are improving. The child is now ready to begin the rehabilitation phase. This usually occurs after 2–7 days. Some children with complications may take longer, whereas others are hungry from the start and can be transferred quickly to F-100. Nevertheless, the transition should be gradual to avoid the risk of heart failure which can occur if children suddenly consume large amounts of feed. Replace the F-75 diet with an equal amount of F-100 for 2 days before increasing the volume offered at each feed (see section 5.2). It is important to note that it is the child's appetite and general condition that determine the phase of treatment and *not* the length of time since admission.

Milk intolerance

Clinically significant milk intolerance is unusual in severely malnourished children. Intolerance should be diagnosed *only* if copious watery diarrhoea occurs promptly after milk-based feeds (e.g. F-100) are begun, the diarrhoea clearly improves when milk intake is reduced or stopped, and it recurs when milk is given again. Other signs include acidic faeces (pH < 5.0) and the presence of increased levels of reducing substances in the faeces. In such cases, the milk should be partially or totally replaced by yoghurt or a commercial lactose-free formula. Before the child is discharged, milk-based feeds should be given again to determine whether the intolerance has resolved.

Recording food intake

The type of feed given, the amounts offered and taken, and the date and time must be recorded accurately after each feed. If the child vomits, the amount lost should be estimated in relation to the size of the feed (e.g. a whole feed, half a feed), and deducted from the total intake. Once a day the energy intake for the past 24 hours should be determined and compared with the child's weight. If the daily intake is less than 80 kcal$_{th}$ or 336 kJ/kg, the amount of feed offered should be increased. If more than 100 kcal$_{th}$ or 420 kJ/kg have been given, the amount of feed offered should be reduced. A sample form for recording food intake is given in Appendix 2.

4.6 Infections

Bacterial infections

Nearly all severely malnourished children have bacterial infections when first admitted to hospital. Many have several infections caused by different organisms. Infection of the lower respiratory tract is especially common. Although signs of infection should be carefully looked for when the child is evaluated, they are often difficult to detect. Unlike well-nourished children, who respond to infection with fever and inflammation, malnourished children with serious infections may only become apathetic or drowsy.

Early treatment of bacterial infections with effective antimicrobials improves the nutritional response to feeding, prevents septic shock and reduces mortality. Because bacterial infections are common and difficult to detect, all children with severe malnutrition should routinely receive broad-spectrum antimicrobial treatment when first admitted for care. Each institution should have a policy on which antimicrobials to use. These are divided into those used for *first-line* treatment, which are given routinely to all severely malnourished children, and those used for *second-line* treatment, which are given when a child is not improving or a specific infection is diagnosed. Although local resistance patterns of important bacterial pathogens and the availability and cost of the antimicrobials will determine the policy, a suggested scheme is given below.

First-line treatment

Children with no apparent signs of infection and no complications should be given cotrimoxazole (25 mg of sulfamethoxazole + 5 mg of trimethoprim/kg) orally twice daily for 5 days.

Children with complications (septic shock, hypoglycaemia, hypothermia, skin infections, respiratory or urinary tract infections, or who appear lethargic or sickly) should be given:

4. Initial treatment

- ampicillin, 50 mg/kg IM or IV every 6 hours for 2 days, followed by amoxicillin, 15 mg/kg orally every 8 hours for 5 days (if amoxicillin is unavailable, give ampicillin, 25 mg/kg orally every 6 hours) *and*
- gentamicin, 7.5 mg/kg IM or IV once daily for 7 days.

Second-line treatment

If the child fails to improve within 48 hours, *add* chloramphenicol, 25 mg/kg IM or IV every 8 hours (or every 6 hours if meningitis is suspected) for 5 days.

Further details of antimicrobial treatment are given in Appendix 6. The duration of treatment depends on the response and nutritional status of the child. Antimicrobials should be continued for at least 5 days. If anorexia still persists after 5 days of treatment, give the child another 5-day course. If anorexia still persists after 10 days of treatment, reassess the child fully. Examine the child for specific infections and potentially resistant organisms, and check that vitamin and mineral supplements have been correctly given.

If specific infections are detected for which additional treatment is needed, for example dysentery, candidiasis, malaria or intestinal helminthiasis, this should also be given (see section 7.3). Tuberculosis is common, but antituberculosis drugs should be given only when tuberculosis is diagnosed (see page 32).

Note: Some institutions routinely give malnourished children metronidazole, 7.5 mg/kg every 8 hours for 7 days, in addition to broad-spectrum antimicrobials. However, the efficacy of this treatment has not been established by clinical trials.

Measles and other viral infections

All malnourished children should receive measles vaccine when admitted to hospital. This protects other children in hospital from catching the disease, which is associated with a high rate of mortality. A second dose of vaccine should be given before discharge.

There is no specific treatment for measles, disseminated herpes or other systemic viral infections. However, most children with these infections develop secondary systemic bacterial infections and septic shock, which should be treated as described in section 4.4. If fever is present (body temperature >39.5 °C or 103 °F), antipyretics should be given.

4.7 Vitamin deficiencies

Vitamin A deficiency

Severely malnourished children are at high risk of developing blindness due to vitamin A deficiency. For this reason a large dose of vitamin A should be given routinely to all malnourished children on day 1, unless there is definitive evidence that a dose has been given during the past month. The dose is as follows:[1] 50 000 International Units (IU) orally for infants <6 months of age, 100 000 IU orally for infants 6–12 months of age and 200 000 IU orally for children >12 months of age. If there are any clinical signs of vitamin A deficiency (e.g. night blindness, conjunctival xerosis with Bitot's spots, corneal xerosis or ulceration, or keratomalacia), a large dose should be given on the first 2 days, followed by a third dose at least 2 weeks later (see Table 10). Oral treatment is preferred, except at the beginning in children with severe anorexia, oedematous malnutrition or septic shock, who should be given IM treatment. For oral treatment, oil-based preparations are

---

[1] The international standard (or reference preparation) of vitamin A has been discontinued. However, the international units for vitamin A are still used extensively, particularly in the labelling of capsules and injectable preparations.

Table 10. Treatment of clinical vitamin A deficiency in children

Timing	Dosage[a,b]
Day 1:	
<6 months of age	50 000 IU
6–12 months of age	100 000 IU
>12 months of age	200 000 IU
Day 2	Same age-specific dose
At least 2 weeks later	Same age-specific dose

[a] For oral administration, preferably in an oil-based preparation, except in children with severe anorexia, oedematous malnutrition or septic shock.
[b] See footnote on page 17.

preferred, but water-miscible formulations may be used if oil-based formulations are not available. Only water-miscible formulations should be used for IM treatment.

Great care must be taken during examination of the eyes, as they easily rupture in children with vitamin A deficiency. The eyes should be examined gently for signs of xerophthalmia, corneal xerosis and ulceration, cloudiness and keratomalacia. If there is ocular inflammation or ulceration, protect the eyes with pads soaked in 0.9% saline. Tetracycline eye drops (1%) should be instilled four times daily until all signs of inflammation or ulceration resolve. Atropine eye drops (0.1%) should also be applied and the affected eye(s) should be bandaged, as scratching with a finger can cause rupture of an ulcerated cornea. More details on the management of vitamin A deficiency are given elsewhere (5, 6).

Other vitamin deficiencies

All malnourished children should receive 5 mg of folic acid orally on day 1 and then 1 mg orally per day thereafter. Many malnourished children are also deficient in riboflavin, ascorbic acid, pyridoxine, thiamine and the fat-soluble vitamins D, E and K. All diets should be fortified with these vitamins by adding the vitamin mix (see Appendix 4).

4.8 Very severe anaemia

If the haemoglobin concentration is less than 40 g/l or the packed-cell volume is less than 12%, the child has very severe anaemia, which can cause heart failure. Children with very severe anaemia need a blood transfusion. Give 10 ml of packed red cells or whole blood per kg of body weight *slowly* over 3 hours. Where testing for HIV and viral hepatitis B is not possible, transfusion should be given only when the haemoglobin concentration falls below 30 g/l (or packed-cell volume below 10%), or when there are signs of life-threatening heart failure. Do *not* give iron during the initial phase of treatment, as it can have toxic effects and may reduce resistance to infection.

4.9 Congestive heart failure

This is usually a complication of overhydration (especially when an IV infusion or standard ORS solution is given), very severe anaemia, blood or plasma transfusion, or giving a diet with a high sodium content. The first sign of heart failure is fast breathing (50 breaths per minute or more if the child is aged 2 months up to 12 months; 40 breaths per minute or more if the child is aged 12 months up to 5 years). Later signs are respiratory distress, a rapid pulse, engorgement of the jugular vein, cold hands and feet, and cyanosis of the fingertips and under the tongue. Heart failure must be differentiated from respiratory infection and septic shock, which usually occur within 48 hours of admission, whereas heart failure usually occurs somewhat later.

When heart failure is caused by fluid overload, the following measures[1] should be taken:

1. Stop *all* oral intake and IV fluids; the treatment of heart failure takes precedence over feeding the child. No fluid should be given until the heart failure is improved, even if this takes 24–48 hours.
2. Give a diuretic IV.[2] The most appropriate choice is furosemide (1 mg/kg).
3. Do not give digitalis unless the diagnosis of heart failure is unequivocal (jugular venous pressure is elevated) *and* the plasma potassium level is normal. In that case, 5 µg/kg of body weight of digoxin may be given IV as a single dose, or orally, if the IV preparation is not available.

4.10 Dermatosis of kwashiorkor

This is characterized by hypo- or hyperpigmentation, shedding of the skin in scales or sheets, and ulceration of the skin of the perineum, groin, limbs, behind the ears and armpits. There may be widespread weeping skin lesions which easily become infected. Spontaneous resolution occurs as nutrition improves. Atrophy of the skin in the perineum leads to severe diaper dermatitis, especially if the child has diarrhoea. The diaper area should be left uncovered. If the diaper area becomes colonized with *Candida* spp., it should be treated with nystatin ointment or cream (100 000 IU (1 g)) twice daily for 2 weeks and the child should be given oral nystatin (100 000 IU four times daily). In other affected areas, application of zinc and castor oil ointment, petroleum jelly or paraffin gauze dressings helps to relieve pain and prevent infection. The zinc supplement contained in the mineral mix is particularly important in these children, as they are usually severely deficient.

Bathe the affected areas in 1% potassium permanganate solution for 10–15 minutes daily. This dries the lesions, helps to prevent loss of serum, and inhibits infection. Polyvidone iodine, 10% ointment, can also be used. It should be used sparingly, however, if the lesions are extensive, as there is significant systemic absorption.

All children with kwashiorkor-related dermatosis should receive systemic antibiotics (see section 4.6).

---

[1] There is no reported experience in malnourished children of angiotensin-converting enzyme inhibitors or other drugs used to treat congestive heart failure.
[2] Diuretics should *never* be used to reduce oedema in malnourished children.

5.
Rehabilitation

The child is deemed to have entered the rehabilitation phase *when his or her appetite has returned.* A child who is being fed by NG tube is *not* considered ready to enter the rehabilitation phase.

5.1 Principles of management

The principal tasks during the rehabilitation phase are:

— to encourage the child to eat as much as possible;
— to re-initiate and/or encourage breastfeeding as necessary;
— to stimulate emotional and physical development; and
— to prepare the mother or carer to continue to look after the child after discharge.

The child should remain in hospital for the first part of the rehabilitation phase. When *all* the criteria in the box below have been met (usually 2–3 weeks after admission), the child can be transferred to a nutrition rehabilitation centre.

Criteria for transfer to a nutrition rehabilitation centre
- Eating well
- Mental state has improved: smiles, responds to stimuli, interested in surroundings
- Sits, crawls, stands or walks (depending on age)
- Normal temperature (36.5–37.5 °C)
- No vomiting or diarrhoea
- No oedema
- Gaining weight: >5 g/kg of body weight per day for 3 successive days

---

5.2 Nutritional rehabilitation

The most important determinant of the rate of recovery is the amount of energy consumed. However, at the start of the rehabilitation phase, the child is still deficient in protein and various micronutrients, including potassium, magnesium, iron and zinc. These must also be given in increased amounts. Infants under 24 months can be fed exclusively on liquid or semi-liquid formulas. It is usually appropriate to introduce solid foods for older children.

Feeding children under 24 months

During rehabilitation, F-100 diet should be given every 4 hours, night and day. Transition to the rehabilitation phase involves increasing the amount of diet given at each feed by 10 ml (e.g. if the first feed is 60 ml, the second should be 70 ml, the third 80 ml, and so on) until the child refuses to finish the feed.

When a feed is not finished, the same amount should be offered at the next feed. If that feed is finished, the amount offered for the following feed should be increased by 10 ml. Continue this process until some food is left after most feeds. The amount being offered should then be dispensed for the child at each feed on subsequent days. The amounts of each feed offered and taken should be recorded on the feeding chart (Appendix 2) and any food not taken should be discarded; *never* reuse it for the next feed. During rehabilitation most children take between 150 and 220 kcal$_{th}$/kg (630–920 kJ/kg) per day. If intake is below 130 kcal$_{th}$ or 540 kJ/kg per day, the child is failing to respond (see section 7).

The attitude of those feeding the child is crucial to success. Sufficient time must be spent with the child to enable him or her to finish each feed. The child must be actively encouraged to eat while sitting comfortably on the mother's or nurse's lap. Children must *never* be left alone to "take what they want".

During the first few days of rehabilitation, children with oedema may not gain weight, despite an adequate intake. This is because oedema fluid is being lost while tissue is being restored. Thus, progress in these children is seen as decreased oedema rather than rapid weight gain. If the child is neither gaining weight nor showing decreased oedema, or if there is increasing oedema, the child is failing to respond (see section 7).

F-100 should be continued until the child achieves –1 SD (90%) of the median NCHS/WHO reference values for weight-for-height (see Appendix 1). When this occurs appetite diminishes and increasing amounts of food are left uneaten. The child is now ready for the discharge phase of treatment.

Feeding children over 24 months

Children over 24 months can also be successfully treated with increasing quantities of F-100; it is not essential to use a different diet. This has practical value in refugee camps where it is important to keep the number of different diets to a minimum. For most older children, however, it is appropriate to introduce solid food, especially for those who want a mixed diet. Most traditional mixed diets have a lower energy content than F-100. They are also relatively deficient in minerals, particularly potassium and magnesium, and contain substances which inhibit the absorption of zinc, copper and iron. Moreover, the diets are usually deficient in various vitamins. Thus, local foods should be fortified to increase their content of energy, minerals and vitamins. Oil should be added to increase the energy content, and the mineral and vitamin mixes used in F-100 should be added after cooking (see section 4.5 and Appendix 4). Other ingredients, such as dried skimmed milk, may also be added to increase the protein and mineral content. The energy content of mixed diets should be *at least* 1 kcal$_{th}$ or 4.2 kJ/g.

To avoid the effects of food substances which reduce the absorption of minerals, F-100 should be given between feeds of the mixed diet. For example, if the mixed diet is given three times daily, F-100 should also be given three times daily, making six feeds a day. Water intake is not usually a problem in children over 2 years because they can ask for it when they are thirsty.

At the beginning of rehabilitation, the children should be fed every 4 hours, day and night (six feeds per 24 hours). When they are growing well and are no longer at risk of developing hypothermia or hypoglycaemia, one of the night-time feeds can be omitted, making five feeds per 24 hours. This allows the child longer undisturbed sleep and makes it much easier to manage the child as a day-patient. It is also less taxing for those caring for the child.

Folic acid and iron

Nearly all severely malnourished children have anaemia and should be given supplementary folic acid and iron. They should also continue to receive the vitamin and mineral mixes in their food throughout rehabilitation.

Iron should *never* be given during the initial phase of treatment, but must be given during the rehabilitation phase. It should only be given orally, *never* by injection.

Children with moderate or severe anaemia should be given elemental iron, 3 mg/kg per day in two divided doses, up to a maximum of 60 mg daily, for 3 months (7). It is preferable to give iron supplements between meals using a liquid preparation.

All children must be given 5 mg of folic acid on day 1 and then 1 mg per day thereafter.

Assessing progress

The child should be weighed daily and the weight plotted on a graph (see Fig. 1 and Appendix 2). It is useful to mark the point that is equivalent to −1 SD (90%) of the median NCHS/WHO reference values for weight-for-height on the graph, which is the target weight for discharge. The usual weight gain is about 10–15 g/kg per day. A child who does not gain *at least* 5 g/kg per day for 3 consecutive days is failing to respond to treatment (see section 7). With high-energy feeding, most severely malnourished children reach their target weight for discharge after 2–4 weeks.

5.3 Emotional and physical stimulation

Severely malnourished children have delayed mental and behavioural development, which, if not treated, can become the most serious long-term result of malnutrition. Emotional and physical stimulation through play programmes that start during rehabilitation and continue after discharge can substantially reduce the risk of permanent mental retardation and emotional impairment.

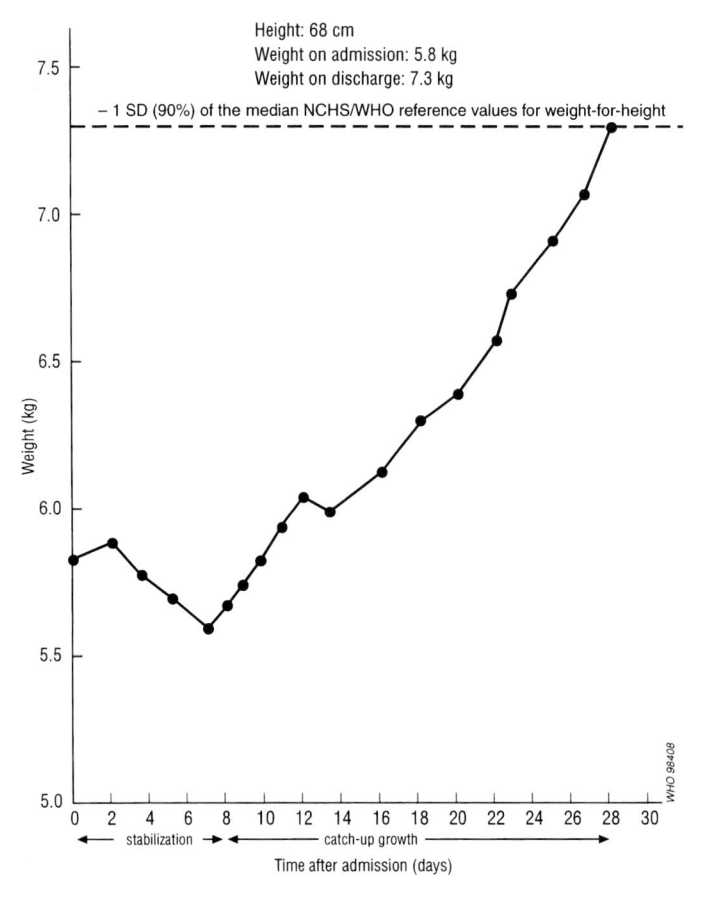

Fig. 1. An example of a weight chart for a severely malnourished boy

Care must be taken to avoid sensory deprivation. The child's face must not be covered; the child must be able to see and hear what is happening around him or her. The child should *never* be wrapped or tied to prevent him or her moving around in the cot.

It is essential that the mother (or carer) be with her child in hospital and at the nutrition rehabilitation centre, and that she be encouraged to feed, hold, comfort and play with her child as much as possible. The number of other adults who interact with the child should be as few as possible. Each adult should talk, smile and show affection towards the child. Medical procedures, such as venepuncture, should be done by the most skilled person available, preferably out of earshot and sight of the other children. Immediately after any unpleasant procedure the child should be held and comforted.

The environment

The austerity of a traditional hospital has no place in the treatment of malnourished children. Rooms should be brightly coloured, with decorations that interest children. Colourful mobiles should be hung over every cot, if possible. The staff should wear normal clothing rather than uniforms. Brightly coloured aprons may be used to protect their clothing. A radio can provide background music. The atmosphere in the ward should be relaxed, cheerful and welcoming.

Toys should always be available in the child's cot and room, as well as in the play area; they should be changed frequently. Toys should be safe, washable and appropriate for the child's age and level of development. Inexpensive toys made from cardboard boxes, plastic bottles, tin cans and similar materials are best, because mothers can copy them. Examples of suitable toys are described in Appendix 7.

Play activities

Malnourished children need interaction with other children during rehabilitation. After the initial phase of treatment, the child should spend prolonged periods with other children on large play mats, and with the mother or a play guide. The child can also be fed in the play area. These activities do not increase the risk of cross-infection appreciably and the benefit for the child is substantial.

One person, usually a nurse or volunteer, should be responsible for developing a curriculum of play activities and for leading the play sessions. Activities should be selected to develop both motor and language skills, and new activities and materials should be introduced regularly. One aim should be to play with each child, individually, for 15–30 minutes each day, in addition to informal group play. A sample curriculum of play activities, arranged by level of development, is provided in Appendix 8. Mothers can be trained to supervise play sessions.

Learning through play should be fun for children. A child's efforts to perform a task should always be praised and never criticized. When a child is taught a skill, the nurse or volunteer should demonstrate the skill first, then help the child do it, and finally let the child do it alone. This sequence should be repeated until the child has mastered the skill.

Physical activities

Physical activities promote the development of essential motor skills and may also enhance growth during rehabilitation. For those children who are unable to move, passive limb movements and splashing in a warm bath are helpful. For other children, play should include such activities as rolling on a mattress, running after and tossing a ball, climbing stairs, and walking. The duration and intensity of physical activities should increase as the child's nutritional status and general condition improve. If there is sufficient space, an outdoor playground should be developed.

5.4 Teaching parents how to prevent malnutrition from recurring

All parents should know how to prevent malnutrition from recurring. Before the child is discharged, ensure that the parents or carers understand the causes of malnutrition and how to prevent its recurrence, including correct feeding and continuing to stimulate the child's mental and emotional development. They must also know how to treat, or obtain treatment for, diarrhoea and other infections, and understand the importance of regular (every 6 months) treatment for intestinal parasites. The parents have much to learn; teaching them should not be left until a few days before the child is discharged.

The mother (or carer) should spend as much time as possible at the nutrition rehabilitation centre with her child. This may be facilitated by providing the mother with money for transportation and meals. The mother, in turn, should help prepare her child's food, and feed and look after her child. A rotation of mothers may also be organized to help with general activities on the ward, including play, cooking, feeding, bathing and changing the children, under supervision. This will enable each mother to learn how to care for her child at home; she will also feel that she is contributing to the work of the centre. Teaching of mothers should include regular sessions at which important parenting skills are demonstrated and practised. Each mother should be taught the play activities that are appropriate for her child, so that she and others in the family can continue to make toys and play with the child after discharge.

The staff must be friendly and treat the mothers as partners in the care of the children. A mother should never be scolded, blamed for her child's problems, humiliated or made to feel unwelcome. Moreover, helping, teaching, counselling and befriending the mother are an essential part of the long-term treatment of the child.

5.5 Preparation for discharge

During rehabilitation, preparations should be made to ensure that the child is fully reintegrated into the family and community after discharge. As the child's home is the environment in which severe malnutrition developed, the family must be carefully prepared to prevent its recurrence. If possible, the child's home should be visited by a social worker or nurse before discharge to ensure that adequate home care can be provided. If the child is abandoned or conditions at the child's home are unsuitable, often because of death or absence of a carer, a foster home should be sought.

Criteria for discharge

A child may be considered to have recovered and be ready for discharge when the child's weight-for-height has reached −1 SD (90%) of the median NCHS/WHO reference values (see Appendix 1). To achieve this goal, it is essential that the child receives as many meals as possible per day. In some instances, a child may be discharged before he or she has reached the target weight-for-height for discharge; however, since the child is not yet recovered, he or she will need continuing care (as an outpatient). To ensure that relapse does not occur, it is important that *all* the criteria listed in Table 11 have been met before the child is discharged.

Appropriate diets

During rehabilitation the child should be fed at least five times daily. After reaching −1 SD of the median NCHS/WHO reference values, the child should be fed at least three times daily at home. Adjustment to this change in frequency of feeding should take place under supervision before discharge. This is done by gradually reducing and eventually stopping the supplementary feeds of F-100 and adding or increasing the mixed diet until the child is eating as he or she will at home.

5. Rehabilitation

Table 11. Criteria for discharge from non-residential care

	Criteria
Child	Weight-for-height has reached −1 SD (90%) of NCHS/WHO median reference values
	Eating an adequate amount of a nutritious diet that the mother can prepare at home
	Gaining weight at a normal or increased rate
	All vitamin and mineral deficiencies have been treated
	All infections and other conditions have been or are being treated, including anaemia, diarrhoea, intestinal parasitic infections, malaria, tuberculosis and otitis media
	Full immunization programme started
Mother or carer	Able and willing to look after the child
	Knows how to prepare appropriate foods and to feed the child
	Knows how to make appropriate toys and to play with the child
	Knows how to give home treatment for diarrhoea, fever and acute respiratory infections, and how to recognize the signs that mean she must seek medical assistance
Health worker	Able to ensure follow-up of the child and support for the mother

Before discharge, the mother (or carer) must practise preparing the recommended foods and feeding them to the child. It is essential that the mother demonstrates that she is able and willing to do these tasks, and that she understands the importance of continued correct feeding for her child. Appropriate mixed diets are the same as those normally recommended for a healthy child. They should provide at least 110 $kcal_{th}$ or 460 kJ/kg per day and also sufficient vitamins and minerals to support continued growth. Breast-feeding should be continued; animal milk is also an important source of energy and protein. Solid foods should include a well-cooked staple cereal, to which vegetable oil should be added (5–10 ml for each 100 g serving) to enrich its energy content. The cereal should be soft and mashed; for infants use a thick pap. A variety of well-cooked vegetables, including orange and dark-green leafy ones, should be given. If possible, include fruit, meat, eggs or fish. The mother should be encouraged to give the child extra food between meals.

Immunization

Before discharge, the child should be immunized in accordance with national guidelines. The mother should be informed of where and when to bring the child for any required booster doses.

Planning follow-up

Before discharge, make an appointment to see the child 1 week after discharge. Follow-up visits should preferably take place at a special clinic for malnourished children, not at a general paediatric clinic.

If possible, arrange for a health worker or field nurse trained to provide practical advice on health and nutrition to visit the family at home. Also arrange for a social worker to visit the family, in order to find a way of solving the family's social and economic problems.

6. Follow-up

Although much improved at the time of discharge, the child usually remains stunted and mental development is delayed. Management of these conditions and preventing the recurrence of severe malnutrition requires sustained improvement in feeding of the child and in other parenting skills. Planned follow-up of the child at regular intervals after discharge is essential. This should include an efficient strategy for tracing children who fail to attend follow-up appointments. Such children are at increased risk of recurrence of malnutrition or of developing other serious illnesses.

As the risk of relapse is greatest soon after discharge, the child should be seen after 1 week, 2 weeks, 1 month, 3 months and 6 months. Provided the child's weight-for-height is no less than −1 SD (90%) of the median NCHS/WHO reference values, progress is considered satisfactory. If a problem is found, visits should be more frequent until it is resolved. After 6 months, visits should be twice yearly until the child is at least 3 years old. Children with frequent problems should remain under supervision longer. The mother should know the location and regular opening hours of the nearest nutrition clinic and be encouraged to bring her child without an appointment if the child is ill or a previous appointment was missed.

At each visit the mother should be asked about the child's recent health, feeding practices and play activities. The child should be examined, weighed and measured, and the results recorded (see Appendix 2). Any needed vaccine should be given. Training of the mother should focus on areas that need to be strengthened, especially feeding practices, and mental and physical stimulation of the child. Attention should also be given to feeding practices for other children in the family, and for pregnant or lactating women, as these are likely to be inadequate. If vitamins or medicines are needed, they should be provided.

7.
Failure to respond to treatment

7.1 General principles

When the treatment guidelines in this manual are followed, a severely malnourished child without complications should show definite signs of improvement within a few days and should continue to improve thereafter. Failure to achieve initial improvement at the expected rate is termed *primary failure to respond*, whereas deterioration of the child's condition, when a satisfactory response has been established, is termed *secondary failure to respond*.

A child who meets any of the criteria in Table 12 should be diagnosed as *failing to respond*. When this diagnosis is made it is essential that practices in the treatment unit are carefully reviewed and the child is thoroughly re-evaluated. The objective is to identify the cause for failure to respond and to correct the problem by making specific changes to practices in the unit or to the child's treatment. Treatment should never be changed blindly; this is more likely to be harmful than to help the child. The most frequent causes of failure to respond are listed in the box below and considered in sections 7.2–7.3.

Frequent causes of failure to respond

Problems with the treatment facility:
- Poor environment for malnourished children
- Insufficient or inadequately trained staff
- Inaccurate weighing machines
- Food prepared or given incorrectly

Problems of individual children:
- Insufficient food given
- Vitamin or mineral deficiency
- Malabsorption of nutrients
- Rumination
- Infections, especially diarrhoea, dysentery, otitis media, pneumonia, tuberculosis, urinary tract infection, malaria, intestinal helminthiasis and HIV/AIDS
- Serious underlying disease

7.2 Problems with the treatment facility

Type of facility

Failure to respond is more likely when a malnourished child is treated in a general paediatric ward than in a special nutrition unit. This is because the risk of cross-infection is increased in a general ward, it is more difficult to provide the necessary care and attention, and staff are less likely to have the essential skills and attitudes for management of malnourished children. Wherever possible, malnourished children should be managed in a special nutrition unit. If this is not possible, they should be treated in a specially designated area of a paediatric ward, by staff specifically trained in the treatment of severe malnutrition.

Table 12. Criteria for failure to respond to treatment

Criteria	Time after admission
Primary failure to respond:	
Failure to regain appetite	Day 4
Failure to start to lose oedema	Day 4
Oedema still present	Day 10
Failure to gain at least 5 g/kg of body weight per day	Day 10
Secondary failure to respond:	
Failure to gain at least 5 g/kg of body weight per day for 3 successive days	During rehabilitation

The special nutrition unit must, however, be well organized. If essential food supplies or medications are not available, weighing scales do not work properly, diagnostic facilities or administrative procedures are inadequate, or there are insufficient trained staff, treatment failure and mortality will be high. An effective management system should ensure careful monitoring of each child, proper training of nurses and auxiliary staff, use of the most experienced staff as supervisors, reliable supplies of drugs and food supplements, and reliable record-keeping.

Staff

Experienced staff (including junior staff) who understand the needs of malnourished children and are familiar with the important details of their management are essential for a well-functioning treatment facility. It is important, therefore, that loss of experienced staff be avoided wherever possible. For this reason, staff of the treatment facility should *not* take part in the routine rotation of staff that is practised in many hospitals. If staff must be changed, this should be done one person at a time so as to minimize disruption of routines in the facility.

The attitude of staff towards a particular child can determine whether treatment of the child will succeed or fail. If staff believe that a child is beyond helping, they may give less attention to the child. Such children often fail to respond to treatment, which seems to confirm the opinion of the staff. This "clinical prejudice" may be difficult to correct, especially when it reflects the views of the most experienced staff. It is essential that staff are reminded frequently that each child's well-being depends on their efforts and that every child must be given their full attention.

Inaccurate weighing machines

Machines used for weighing children easily become inaccurate and, thus, give misleading information on the progress of children in the facility. Weighing machines must be checked and adjusted daily following a standard procedure. Records of daily checks should be kept. Weighing machines used for preparing food or for measuring the ingredients of the mineral mix should be checked and adjusted weekly.

Problems with preparing or giving food

Standard hygiene practices should be used when storing, preparing and handling food in the kitchen of the hospital or nutrition rehabilitation centre. Hands should be washed with soap after defecation and before food is handled. Foods should be thoroughly cooked and served promptly. Any cooked food that will be stored for more than 2 hours should be refrigerated (after allowing it to cool to room temperature) and re-heated until it is thoroughly hot (and then allowed to cool) before being served. Persons with infections on their hands should not handle food.

Each person involved in preparing food should be checked to ensure that they are following the correct procedures for weighing, measuring, mixing, cooking and storing the food. Observe the feeds being made; check that the recipes are correct and all ingredients are added.

Ensure that sufficient time is allocated to feeding each child and that there are enough staff, day and night, for this task. Remember that feeding a malnourished child takes more time and patience than feeding a normal child. If it is assumed that it takes about 15 minutes to feed each child and that food is given every 3 hours, one person is needed, day and night, to feed 12 children. When food is given every 2 hours, more staff are needed. If there are not enough staff, treatment of a child may fail because insufficient time is taken for feeding. Having the mother help with feeding her child can relieve this situation.

7.3 Problems with individual children

Feeding

Is enough food being given?

Recalculate the food requirement for the child. Ensure that the correct amount is being offered at the required times, and that the amount taken by the child is measured and recorded accurately. Observe the measuring and giving of food. Check the calculation of the daily energy intake of the child. Review the feeding guidelines in sections 4.5 and 5.2, giving particular attention to feeding during the night, as this is often done less well than during the day.

A child treated at a nutrition rehabilitation centre may fail to respond because the feeds provided at home are too few or too small, or incorrectly prepared. Such failures usually indicate that the family was not adequately counselled initially. If, despite corrective measures, the child fails to respond, the child should be readmitted to hospital.

Are sufficient vitamins and minerals being given?

Nutrient deficiency can result from the increased requirements related to the synthesis of new tissue during rapid growth. When this happens, there is usually an initial period of rapid growth, after which growth slows or stops even though food intake is adequate. Deficiencies of potassium, magnesium, zinc, copper or iron may be responsible. Diets are often deficient in these minerals and commercial vitamin and mineral preparations do not provide them in sufficient amounts for severely malnourished children. This problem can be avoided by ensuring that the mineral and vitamin mixes described in Appendix 4 are added to the child's food every day.

Is the child ruminating?

Rumination is a condition that occurs in up to 10% of severely malnourished, emotionally impaired children. It should be suspected when a child eats well, but fails to gain weight. Children with this condition regurgitate food from the stomach into the mouth, and then vomit part of it and swallow the rest. This usually happens when they are ignored, so it may not be observed. Such children are usually thought to have vomiting without diarrhoea because they often smell of vomit, and may have vomit-stained clothes or bedding. They are often unusually alert and suspicious, may make stereotyped chewing movements, and do not appear distressed by vomiting.

Rumination is best treated by staff members who have experience with this problem and give special attention to the child. They need to show disapproval whenever the child begins to ruminate, without being intimidating, and to encourage other less harmful behaviours.

Infection

Unrecognized infections are a frequent cause of failure to respond. Those most often overlooked include pneumonia, urinary tract infection, otitis media and tuberculosis. Others include malaria, dengue, viral hepatitis B and HIV infection. Children who fail to respond to treatment should be investigated for infection as follows:

1. Examine the child carefully. Measure the child's temperature, pulse rate and respiration rate every 3 hours. As already mentioned, infection in a malnourished child often causes hypothermia.
2. If possible, obtain a chest X-ray. Examine the urine for pus cells. Examine and culture the sputum or a tracheal aspirate for tubercle bacilli. Examine the stool for signs of blood, *Giardia* trophozoites or cysts and *Strongyloides stercoralis* larvae, and culture for bacterial pathogens. Culture the blood and test for the presence of viral hepatitis B and malaria. Examine and culture the cerebrospinal fluid.

Specific infections are discussed below.

Persistent diarrhoea

This is diarrhoea that occurs every day for at least 14 days. Weight loss is common. ReSoMal should be given to prevent or treat dehydration (see section 4.4). If the stool contains visible blood, treat the child with an oral antimicrobial that is effective against most local strains of *Shigella* (see treatment guidelines for dysentery below). If cysts or trophozoites of *Giardia* are found in the stool, treat the child with metronidazole, 5 mg/kg orally three times daily for 5 days. Blind antimicrobial therapy, however, is ineffective and should not be given. Every child with persistent diarrhoea should be examined for non-intestinal infections, such as pneumonia, sepsis, urinary tract infection and otitis media. Antimicrobial treatment of these infections should follow standard guidelines. Antidiarrhoeal drugs should *never* be used. Such drugs are not effective in children and some may be dangerous.

Feeding guidelines are the same as for severe malnutrition. Breast-feeding should be continued as often and for as long as the child wants. Milk intolerance is rare when the recommended feeding guidelines for malnutrition are followed. However, if it occurs (see section 4.5), replace the animal milk with yoghurt or a commercial lactose-free formula. Persistent diarrhoea usually resolves when the child begins to gain weight.

Further details of treatment of diarrhoea are available elsewhere (*8*).

Dysentery

This is diarrhoea with visible blood in the stool. *Shigella* is the most frequent cause, especially of cases that are severe. Treatment is with an oral antibiotic to which most local strains of *Shigella* are sensitive. Unfortunately, the choice of antimicrobials for treatment of shigellosis has narrowed considerably in recent years as the prevalence of antimicrobial resistance has increased. Resistance to ampicillin and cotrimoxazole (sulfamethoxazole + trimethoprim), formerly the drugs of choice, is now widespread. Nevertheless, cotrimoxazole (25 mg of sulfamethoxazole + 5 mg of trimethoprim/kg orally twice daily for 5 days) and, in a few areas, ampicillin (25 mg/kg four times daily for 5 days) may still be effective against most endemic strains. Nalidixic acid (15 mg/kg four times daily for 5 days), which was formerly reserved for the treatment of resistant cases of shigellosis, is now the drug of choice in many areas. If there is no improvement (less blood in the stool or passage of fewer stools) after 2 days, the antibiotic should be changed to another to which local strains of *Shigella* are sensitive (see Appendix 6). Accordingly, health facilities in areas where there is a high incidence of bloody diarrhoea should ensure that several antimicrobials known to be effective against most local strains of *Shigella* spp. are kept in stock.

Amoebiasis. Amoebiasis can cause dysentery, liver abscess and other systemic complications, but is rare in children under 5 years. Treatment for amoebiasis should be given when motile trophozoites of *Entamoeba histolytica* containing ingested erythrocytes are found in a fresh stool sample or when bloody diarrhoea continues after successive treatment with two antibiotics that are usually effective for *Shigella*. The finding of amoebic cysts in the stools is not sufficient for a diagnosis of amoebiasis. Treatment is with metronidazole oral suspension, 10 mg/kg three times daily for 5–10 days (see Appendix 6).

Giardiasis. Intestinal infection with *Giardia* is common and usually has no adverse effect on well-nourished children. However, in severely malnourished children, treatment for giardiasis should be given when cysts or trophozoites of *Giardia* are seen in the stool. Treatment is with metronidazole, 5 mg/kg orally three times daily for 5 days (see Appendix 6).

Further details of treatment for children with dysentery are available elsewhere (9).

Otitis media

Otitis media occurs frequently in children, often in connection with hospital-acquired upper respiratory infection. There are no specific clinical signs, except when the eardrum has ruptured, causing drainage from the ear. The diagnosis usually requires examination of the ears with an otoscope, looking for loss of the tympanic light reflex or perforation of the eardrum. Typical signs of inflammation may not be present. Treatment is with cotrimoxazole (25 mg of sulfamethoxazole + 5 mg of trimethoprim/kg twice daily), ampicillin (25 mg/kg four times daily) or amoxicillin (15 mg/kg three times daily) for 5 days (see Appendix 6). A cotton wick should be used to dry any drainage from the ear.

Pneumonia

Pneumonia is manifested by fast breathing and, sometimes, chest indrawing. Cough, crackly breath sounds and abnormalities on chest X-ray are frequently absent. The cut-off for fast breathing is 50 times per minute or more if the child is aged 2–12 months, or 40 times per minute or more if the child is aged 12 months to 5 years. Children with fast breathing should be diagnosed as having pneumonia and given an oral antimicrobial for 5 days. Cotrimoxazole (sulfamethoxazole + trimethoprim), ampicillin or amoxicillin is usually effective (see above). Children with fast breathing and chest indrawing should be treated with benzylpenicillin, 50 000 IU/kg IM four times daily for at least 5 days, until they improve, and then with oral ampicillin or amoxicillin (see above). Oxygen should also be given if the breathing rate is over 70 breaths per minute.

For further details of treatment for children with otitis media and pneumonia, see reference *10.*

Urinary tract infections

Urinary tract infections occur frequently, with a similar incidence in boys and girls. Such infections are usually asymptomatic and are diagnosed using dip-stick tests or by finding large numbers of leukocytes on microscopic examination of fresh urine (at least 10 leukocytes per microscope field (X40 magnification)). Cotrimoxazole (25 mg of sulfamethoxazole + 5 mg of trimethoprim/kg twice daily for 5 days) is usually effective.

Alternatively, ampicillin (25 mg/kg four times daily for 5 days) can be given (see Appendix 6).

Skin infections

Bacterial infections. These include pustules, impetigo, infected fissures (especially behind the ears) and indolent ulcers. Treatment should include washing the affected area with soap and water, and gently removing debris and crusts by soaking in warm saline or clean warm water. Dry the child carefully and apply polyvidone iodine, 10% ointment, or chlorhexidine, 5% lotion, to the affected area. Widespread superficial and deep-seated infections should be treated with benzylpenicillin, 50 000 IU/kg IM four times daily for at least 10 days. If abscesses are present, they should be drained surgically.

Candidiasis. Oral candidiasis causes creamy-white lesions in the mouth and may be painful, making feeding difficult. The diagnosis is confirmed by the presence of typical yeast forms on Gram staining of scrapings from the lesion. Candidiasis can also involve the oesophagus, stomach, rectum and moist tissues (e.g. axillae, groin). In systemic candidiasis, the respiratory tract and blood may be involved. Nystatin oral suspension, 100 000 IU four times daily is recommended for oral, oesophageal and rectal candidiasis. Nystatin cream (100 000 IU (1 g)) should be applied to affected areas of skin twice daily for 2 weeks. Children over 2 years with systemic candidiasis should be given ketoconazole, 5 mg/kg orally daily until remission is obtained.

Scabies. Scabies is caused by a mite that burrows superficially into the skin and causes intense itching; the scratched lesions often become secondarily infected. Lindane, 0.3% lotion, should be applied to affected areas once daily for 2 days. If this is not available, benzyl benzoate, 25% lotion, may be used. Although cheaper, it is more irritating; it should be avoided in malnourished children, unless there is no alternative available. Family members should also be treated to prevent infestation or reinfestation.

Tuberculosis

Tuberculosis is an important cause of failure to respond. The diagnosis is made by chest X-ray and examination or culture of sputum or tracheal secretions. Occasionally, typical tuberculous lesions can be seen in the fundus of the eye. The Mantoux test is often negative owing to anergy, but may become positive as the child's nutritional status improves.

Antituberculosis drugs should be given only when tuberculosis is diagnosed, and treatment should follow guidelines published by WHO (*11*) or national guidelines. Children with HIV infection are at increased risk of tuberculosis and should be treated if tuberculosis is suspected. As the recommended drugs are hepatotoxic, they should be used with caution in any child with an enlarged or tender liver. The recommended treatment schedule is described in Appendix 6.

Helminthiasis

Ascariasis, hookworm infection and trichuriasis. Infection with *Ascaris lumbricoides* (roundworm), *Ancylostoma duodenale* or *Necator americanus* (hookworm), and *Trichuris trichiura* (whipworm) is common in children who play outside. Whipworm infections can cause dysentery, anaemia and, occasionally, prolapse of the rectum. Hookworm infections can cause severe anaemia. Treatment of these infections should be delayed until the rehabilitation phase of treatment for severe malnutrition. Albendazole (400 mg in a single dose) and mebendazole (100 mg twice daily for 3 days for inpatient treatment or 500 mg in a single dose for outpatient treatment) are both effective in children over 2 years. If these drugs are not available or the child is under 2 years, hookworm can be treated with pyrantel (10 mg/kg in a single dose) and ascariasis with pyrantel or piperazine. Piperazine is also effective in whipworm infections. Children aged 2–12 years should be given 75 mg/kg of piperazine in a single dose to a maximum of 2.5 g, while those under 2 years should receive 50 mg/kg in a single dose administered under medical supervision (see Appendix 6).

Strongyloidiasis. Infection with *Strongyloides stercoralis* is also common in children who play outside. The diagnosis is made by detecting typical larvae in the faeces. In patients whose immune systems are depressed by disease, the larvae may become widely disseminated, giving rise to life-threatening pulmonary, cerebral and hepatic complications. Albendazole is the drug of choice for children over 2 years; 400 mg should be given in a single oral dose. If albendazole is unavailable or the child is under 2 years, ivermectin should be given; the dosage is 200 µg/kg in a single oral dose. Tiabendazole is effective, but causes severe anorexia, which is dangerous for malnourished children.

Malaria

Malaria is diagnosed by microscopic examination of a blood smear for malarial parasites. Malaria often appears during the rehabilitation phase of treatment for malnutrition. Malnourished children with malaria should receive a full course of antimalarial therapy with the dosage based on body weight.

Non-falciparum malaria. Infections with *Plasmodium ovale, P. malariae* or susceptible forms of *P. vivax* may be treated with chloroquine. The total daily dose of chloroquine is 25 mg of base/kg orally given over 3 days as follows (see Appendix 6):

- Days 1 and 2: 10 mg of base/kg in a single dose
- Day 3: 5 mg of base/kg in a single dose.

Falciparum malaria. A single drug should be given following national recommendations. Drugs that may be recommended for children include chloroquine (see above), quinine and pyrimethamine + sulfadoxine. The dose of quinine is 8 mg of base/kg orally every 8 hours for 7 days. The dose of pyrimethamine + sulfadoxine is adjusted according to the body weight of the child as follows:

- 5–10 kg: 12.5 mg + 250 mg orally in a single dose
- 11–20 kg: 25 mg + 500 mg orally in a single dose.

HIV infection and AIDS

Children with acquired immunodeficiency syndrome (AIDS) are likely to present with severe malnutrition. In some countries up to half of the children presenting with severe malnutrition have AIDS. Treatment of malnutrition in children with HIV infection or AIDS is the same as in children who are HIV-negative. Interstitial lymphocytic pneumonia is specifically associated with HIV infection. If findings on X-ray are typical of interstitial lymphocytic pneumonia, an HIV test should be performed. Treatment is with steroids.

Severely malnourished children should *not* be tested routinely for HIV. Knowledge of HIV status plays no role in management of the child, except to diagnose interstitial lymphocytic pneumonia. When an HIV test is done, the results should *not* be revealed to the staff. Otherwise, a positive test may cause them to neglect the child.

Serious underlying disease

Malnutrition may result from unrecognized congenital abnormalities, inborn errors of metabolism, malignancies, immunological diseases and other diseases of the major organs. Examination of a child who fails to respond to treatment should include a search for serious underlying disease. Any problem identified should be treated appropriately;

however, the associated malnutrition should be managed according to the guidelines in this manual.

7.4 Learning from failure

Accurate records should be kept of all children who fail to respond to treatment and of all deaths. These should include, as a minimum, details of the child's age, sex, date of admission, weight-for-height (or length) on admission, principal diagnoses, treatment and, where appropriate, date and time of death, and apparent cause of death. Periodic review of these records can help to identify areas where case management practices should be carefully examined and improved. For example, deaths that occur within the first 2 days are often due to hypoglycaemia, unrecognized or mismanaged septic shock, or other serious infection, whereas deaths that occur after day 2 are often due to heart failure. An increase in deaths occurring at night or at weekends suggests that monitoring and care of children at those times should be reviewed and improved. The objective should be to achieve a case-fatality rate of <5%.

8.
Management of malnutrition in disaster situations and refugee camps

8.1 General considerations

Health workers in disaster situations and refugee camps may have to manage a large number of severely malnourished children. Although the principles of management are the same as in other situations, treatment must follow a routine, rather than an individual, approach. This often requires that a therapeutic feeding centre be established. This is usually necessary when a cluster survey shows over 10% of children aged 6 months to 5 years with low weight-for-height (below −2 SD of the median NCHS/WHO reference values) (*12*).

8.2 Establishing a therapeutic feeding centre

Location and capacity

If possible, the therapeutic feeding centre should be in or near a hospital. It may be located in simple buildings or tents. One centre can serve up to 50 children. If there are more than 50–100 children, a second centre should be established. Each centre should include a special care unit, to provide round-the-clock care during initial treatment, and a day-care unit, to provide care during rehabilitation.

Water supply and sanitation

A minimum of 30 litres of water should be available per child per day. If less than 10 litres of water are available per child per day, the centre will be unable to function. A latrine and a bathing area are required for every 20 persons.

Cooking facilities and supplies

A collective kitchen should be organized and a reliable supply of fuel for cooking ensured. The food requirement should be based on the estimated number of severely malnourished children plus their mothers or carers. Secure storage facilities are required for food and medical supplies.

Staff

Each centre should include, as a minimum, one part-time doctor, three nurses and 10 nursing aides. The mothers or carers of the children may also provide assistance.

8.3 Criteria for enrolment and discharge

The criteria for admission depend on the objectives of the programme and the resources available. In general, children whose weight-for-height is below −3 SD or 70% of the median NCHS/WHO reference values, or who have oedema, should be admitted to the therapeutic feeding centre. Discharge usually takes place when the child's weight-for-height has reached at least −2 SD or 80% (preferably −1.5 SD or 85%) of the NCHS/WHO median reference values on two consecutive weighings, 1 week apart. In some situations the circumference of the mid upper arm (*13*) is used as a criterion for admission. The criteria can be modified in accordance with national guidelines, resources of the centre and capacity for follow-up, but should always be clearly defined.

8.4 Principles of management

The principles of management are the same as in a hospital setting. The doctor should evaluate each child daily. Initial treatment should include vitamins, minerals, anthelminthics (see page 32) and antimicrobials (see section 4.6).

8.5 Evaluation of the therapeutic feeding centre

A medical team should monitor the health and nutritional status of the *entire* population of the refugee camp or disaster area by:

— calculating mean daily mortality rates at weekly intervals;
— monitoring the availability of food, and its macro- and micronutrient content, at monthly intervals; and
— conducting anthropometric (weight and height or length) surveys every 3 months.

The rates of coverage, success and mortality of the centre should be regularly evaluated by the following criteria:

- *Coverage rate*: The number of severely malnourished children enrolled at the centre divided by the total number of severely malnourished children in the population, based on the most recent survey.
- *Recovery rate*: The number of children reaching criteria for discharge divided by the total number of discharges, deaths, defaulters and transfers.
- *Mortality rate*: The number of deaths among children at the centre divided by the total number of children enrolled at the centre.

The interpretation of these figures depends on local conditions, resources and competing health priorities. Most programmes can achieve coverage rates of at least 80%, with recovery rates of >50%, and mortality rates of <15%.

9.
Malnutrition in adolescents and adults

Severe malnutrition occurs as a primary disorder in adolescents and adults in conditions of extreme privation and famine. It also occurs in situations of dependency, for example, in the elderly, those with mental illnesses and emotional problems, and in prisoners. Malnutrition in adolescents and adults is commonly associated with other illnesses, such as chronic infections, intestinal malabsorption, alcohol and drug dependence, liver disease, endocrine and autoimmune diseases, cancer and AIDS. In such cases both the malnutrition and the underlying illness must be treated.

9.1 Principles of management

The physiological changes and principles of management of adolescents and adults with severe malnutrition are the same as those in children. In general, the guidelines for management of children should be followed. There are, however, differences in the classification of malnutrition, the amount of food required and the drug dosages.

Except in famine conditions, adolescents and adults rarely associate wasting or oedema with their diet. As a consequence, they do not believe that altering their diet will help them. Even in famine conditions, they are often very reluctant to eat anything except traditional foods, which they view as perfectly satisfactory. Moreover, the foods they are allowed are often restricted by cultural and religious beliefs. They are often reluctant to take formula feeds unless they can be persuaded that such feeds are a form of medicine. This problem is one of the most difficult aspects of treating adolescents and adults.

9.2 Classification of malnutrition

Adults (over 18 years)

Body mass index

The degree of thinness is assessed using the body mass index (BMI) as the indicator. BMI is defined as the body weight (in kg) divided by the square of the height[1] (in metres). Table 13 gives the BMI cut-off values for defining grades of malnutrition in adults.

When an adult is too ill to stand or has a spinal deformity, the half arm span should be measured. This is the distance from the middle of the sternal notch to the tip of the middle finger with the arm held out horizontally to the side. Both sides should be measured. If there is a discrepancy, the measurements should be repeated and the longest one taken. The height (in metres) can then be calculated as follows:

$$\text{Height} = [0.73 \times (2 \times \text{half arm span})] + 0.43$$

The BMI is then computed from the calculated height and measured weight.

---

[1] Short height, in adults, usually represents chronic malnutrition in childhood. As there is no treatment available, short adult height is mainly of theoretical interest, except that stunted women have an increased risk of complications during delivery and are likely to have low-birth-weight and short children themselves.

Table 13. Classification of malnutrition in adults by body mass index[a]

Body mass index	Nutritional status
≥18.5	Normal
17.0–18.49	Mild malnutrition
16.0–16.99	Moderate malnutrition
<16.0	Severe malnutrition

[a] For further information, see reference *1*.

Oedema

Examine the ankles and lower legs for pitting oedema. If symmetrical oedema is present, its cause must be determined. In addition to malnutrition, causes in adults include pre-eclampsia (in pregnant women), severe proteinuria (nephrotic syndrome), nephritis, acute filariasis (the limb is hot and painful), heart failure and wet beriberi. Non-nutritional causes of oedema can readily be identified by the history, physical examination and urinalysis.

Adults with a BMI below 16.0 or with oedematous malnutrition should be admitted to hospital.

Adolescents (10–18 years)

A WHO Expert Committee has recommended BMI-for-age as the best indicator of thinness for use in adolescence, the cut-off value being <5th percentile[1] (*1*). In that case, or when nutritional oedema exists, malnutrition should be diagnosed. For stunting or low height-for-age, the cut-off value is <3rd percentile or below –2 SD of the median NCHS/WHO reference values.

9.3 History and physical examination

A thorough examination should be conducted to exclude conditions that give rise to secondary malnutrition (see page 37). A careful dietary history should be taken. Blood sugar should be tested to exclude diabetes mellitus.

9.4 Initial treatment

If possible, adolescents and adults should be given the same formula feeds (with added minerals and vitamins) as children (see section 4.5). The initial goal of treatment is to prevent further loss of tissue. The amount of feed given per kg of body weight is much less than for children and decreases with increasing age, reflecting the lower energy requirements of adults. Recommended amounts for different ages are given in Table 14. These amounts will meet all nutrient requirements of adolescents and adults. As most severely malnourished adults are anorexic, the formula is usually given by NG tube during the first few days.

Adults and adolescents are also susceptible to hypothermia and hypoglycaemia. The latter condition is managed as described for children (see section 4.2). They should also be given systemic antibiotics and, except for pregnant women, a single dose of 200 000 IU of vitamin A orally (*6*).

---

[1] Defined as the rank position of an individual on a given reference distribution, stated in terms of what percentage of the group the individual equals or exceeds. Thus an adolescent of a given age whose weight falls in the 5th percentile weighs the same or more than 5% of the reference population of adolescents of the same age.

Table 14. **Dietary requirements for initial treatment of severely malnourished adolescents and adults**

Age (years)	Daily energy requirement[a]		Volume of diet required (ml/kg per hour)	
	(kcal$_{th}$/kg)	(kJ/kg)	F-75	F-100
7–10	75	315	4.2	3.0
11–14	60	250	3.5	2.5
15–18	50	210	2.8	2.0
19–75	40	170	2.2	1.7
>75	35	150	2.0	1.5

[a] Individual needs may vary by up to 30% from these figures.

9.5 Rehabilitation

An improving appetite indicates the beginning of rehabilitation. During rehabilitation it is usual for adolescents and adults to become very hungry, often refusing the formula feed and demanding enormous amounts of solid food. When this happens, a diet should be given that is based on traditional foods, but with added oil, mineral mix and vitamin mix. Provide a wide variety of foods and allow the patients to eat as much as they want. If possible, continue to give the formula feed with the vitamin and mineral mixes between meals and at night. If necessary, present the formula feed as a medicine.

9.6 Criteria for discharge

Adolescents and adults can be discharged when they are eating well and gaining weight, they have a reliable source of nutritious food outside the hospital, and any other health problems have been diagnosed and treatment begun. Adults should continue to receive a supplemented diet as outpatients until their BMI is ⩾18.5; for adolescents, their diets should be supplemented until their BMI-for-age is ⩾5th percentile of the median NCHS/WHO reference values.

9.7 Failure to respond to treatment

Failure to respond to treatment in adults and adolescents is usually due to an unrecognized underlying illness (see page 37), a nutrient deficiency or refusal to follow the treatment regimen.

References

1. *Physical status: the use and interpretation of anthropometry. Report of a WHO Expert Committee.* Geneva, World Health Organization, 1995 (WHO Technical Report Series, No. 854).

2. Waterlow JC. Note on the assessment and classification of protein–energy malnutrition in children. *Lancet*, 1973, i:87–89.

3. Waterlow JC. Classification and definition of protein–calorie malnutrition. *British medical journal*, 1972, 3: 566–569.

4. Gomez F et al. Mortality in second- and third-degree malnutrition. *Journal of tropical pediatrics and African child health*, 1956, 2:77.

5. Sommer A. *Vitamin A deficiency and its consequences. A field guide to detection and control*, 3rd ed. Geneva, World Health Organization, 1995.

6. *Vitamin A supplements: a guide to their use in the treatment and prevention of vitamin A deficiency and xerophthalmia*, 2nd ed. Geneva, World Health Organization, 1997.

7. *Iron deficiency: assessment, prevention and control.* Geneva, World Health Organization, 1998 (unpublished document WHO/NUT/98.6; available on request from Programme of Nutrition, World Health Organization, 1211 Geneva 27, Switzerland).

8. *The treatment of diarrhoea. A manual for physicians and other senior health workers.* Geneva, World Health Organization, 1995 (unpublished document WHO/CDR/95.3; available on request from Division of Child Health and Development, World Health Organization, 1211 Geneva 27, Switzerland).

9. *The management of bloody diarrhoea in young children.* Geneva, World Health Organization, 1994 (unpublished document WHO/CDD/94.49; available on request from Division of Child Health and Development, World Health Organization, 1211 Geneva 27, Switzerland).

10. *Acute respiratory infections in children: case management in small hospitals in developing countries.* Geneva, World Health Organization, 1990 (unpublished document WHO/ARI/90.5; available on request from Distribution and Sales, World Health Organization, 1211 Geneva 27, Switzerland).

11. *Treatment of tuberculosis: guidelines for national programmes*, 2nd ed. Geneva, World Health Organization, 1997 (unpublished document WHO/TB/97.220; available on request from Global Tuberculosis Programme, World Health Organization, 1211 Geneva 27, Switzerland).

12. *The management of nutrition in major emergencies*, 2nd ed. Geneva, World Health Organization, in press.

13. de Onis M, Yip R, Mei Z. The development of MUAC-for-age reference data recommended by a WHO Expert Committee. *Bulletin of the World Health Organization*, 1997, 75:11–18.

Appendix 1

NCHS/WHO normalized reference values for weight-for-height and weight-for-length

Boys' weight (kg)					Length[a] (cm)	Girls' weight (kg)				
−4 SD	−3 SD	−2 SD	−1 SD	Median		Median	−1 SD	−2 SD	−3 SD	−4 SD
1.8	2.1	2.5	2.8	3.1	49	3.3	2.9	2.6	2.2	1.8
1.8	2.2	2.5	2.9	3.3	50	3.4	3.0	2.6	2.3	1.9
1.8	2.2	2.6	3.1	3.5	51	3.5	3.1	2.7	2.3	1.9
1.9	2.3	2.8	3.2	3.7	52	3.7	3.3	2.8	2.4	2.0
1.9	2.4	2.9	3.4	3.9	53	3.9	3.4	3.0	2.5	2.1
2.0	2.6	3.1	3.6	4.1	54	4.1	3.6	3.1	2.7	2.2
2.2	2.7	3.3	3.8	4.3	55	4.3	3.8	3.3	2.8	2.3
2.3	2.9	3.5	4.0	4.6	56	4.5	4.0	3.5	3.0	2.4
2.5	3.1	3.7	4.3	4.8	57	4.8	4.2	3.7	3.1	2.6
2.7	3.3	3.9	4.5	5.1	58	5.0	4.4	3.9	3.3	2.7
2.9	3.5	4.1	4.8	5.4	59	5.3	4.7	4.1	3.5	2.9
3.1	3.7	4.4	5.0	5.7	60	5.5	4.9	4.3	3.7	3.1
3.3	4.0	4.6	5.3	5.9	61	5.8	5.2	4.6	3.9	3.3
3.5	4.2	4.9	5.6	6.2	62	6.1	5.4	4.8	4.1	3.5
3.8	4.5	5.2	5.8	6.5	63	6.4	5.7	5.0	4.4	3.7
4.0	4.7	5.4	6.1	6.8	64	6.7	6.0	5.3	4.6	3.9
4.3	5.0	5.7	6.4	7.1	65	7.0	6.3	5.5	4.8	4.1
4.5	5.3	6.0	6.7	7.4	66	7.3	6.5	5.8	5.1	4.3
4.8	5.5	6.2	7.0	7.7	67	7.5	6.8	6.0	5.3	4.5
5.1	5.8	6.5	7.3	8.0	68	7.8	7.1	6.3	5.5	4.8
5.3	6.0	6.8	7.5	8.3	69	8.1	7.3	6.5	5.8	5.0
5.5	6.3	7.0	7.8	8.5	70	8.4	7.6	6.8	6.0	5.2
5.8	6.5	7.3	8.1	8.8	71	8.6	7.8	7.0	6.2	5.4
6.0	6.8	7.5	8.3	9.1	72	8.9	8.1	7.2	6.4	5.6
6.2	7.0	7.8	8.6	9.3	73	9.1	8.3	7.5	6.6	5.8
6.4	7.2	8.0	8.8	9.6	74	9.4	8.5	7.7	6.8	6.0
6.6	7.4	8.2	9.0	9.8	75	9.6	8.7	7.9	7.0	6.2
6.8	7.6	8.4	9.2	10.0	76	9.8	8.9	8.1	7.2	6.4
7.0	7.8	8.6	9.4	10.3	77	10.0	9.1	8.3	7.4	6.6
7.1	8.0	8.8	9.7	10.5	78	10.2	9.3	8.5	7.6	6.7
7.3	8.2	9.0	9.9	10.7	79	10.4	9.5	8.7	7.8	6.9
7.5	8.3	9.2	10.1	10.9	80	10.6	9.7	8.8	8.0	7.1
7.6	8.5	9.4	10.2	11.1	81	10.8	9.9	9.0	8.1	7.2
7.8	8.7	9.6	10.4	11.3	82	11.0	10.1	9.2	8.3	7.4
7.9	8.8	9.7	10.6	11.5	83	11.2	10.3	9.4	8.5	7.6
8.1	9.0	9.9	10.8	11.7	84	11.4	10.5	9.6	8.7	7.7

SD: standard deviation score (or Z-score). Although the interpretation of a fixed percent-of-median value varies across age and height, and generally the two scales cannot be compared, the approximate percent-of-median values for −1 and −2 SD are 90% and 80% of median, respectively (Gorstein J et al. Issues in the assessment of nutritional status using anthropometry. *Bulletin of the World Health Organization*, 1994, 72:273–283).

[a] Length is measured for children below 85 cm. For children 85 cm or more, height is measured. Recumbent length is on average 0.5 cm greater than standing height; although the difference is of no importance to individual children, a correction may be made by subtracting 0.5 cm from all lengths above 84.9 cm if standing height cannot be measured.

Boys' weight (kg)					Height[a] (cm)	Girls' weight (kg)				
−4 SD	−3 SD	−2 SD	−1 SD	Median		Median	−1 SD	−2 SD	−3 SD	−4 SD
7.8	8.9	9.9	11.0	12.1	85	11.8	10.8	9.7	8.6	7.6
7.9	9.0	10.1	11.2	12.3	86	12.0	11.0	9.9	8.8	7.7
8.1	9.2	10.3	11.5	12.6	87	12.3	11.2	10.1	9.0	7.9
8.3	9.4	10.5	11.7	12.8	88	12.5	11.4	10.3	9.2	8.1
8.4	9.6	10.7	11.9	13.0	89	12.7	11.6	10.5	9.3	8.2
8.6	9.8	10.9	12.1	13.3	90	12.9	11.8	10.7	9.5	8.4
8.8	9.9	11.1	12.3	13.5	91	13.2	12.0	10.8	9.7	8.5
8.9	10.1	11.3	12.5	13.7	92	13.4	12.2	11.0	9.9	8.7
9.1	10.3	11.5	12.8	14.0	93	13.6	12.4	11.2	10.0	8.8
9.2	10.5	11.7	13.0	14.2	94	13.9	12.6	11.4	10.2	9.0
9.4	10.7	11.9	13.2	14.5	95	14.1	12.9	11.6	10.4	9.1
9.6	10.9	12.1	13.4	14.7	96	14.3	13.1	11.8	10.6	9.3
9.7	11.0	12.4	13.7	15.0	97	14.6	13.3	12.0	10.7	9.5
9.9	11.2	12.6	13.9	15.2	98	14.9	13.5	12.2	10.9	9.6
10.1	11.4	12.8	14.1	15.5	99	15.1	13.8	12.4	11.1	9.8
10.3	11.6	13.0	14.4	15.7	100	15.4	14.0	12.7	11.3	9.9
10.4	11.8	13.2	14.6	16.0	101	15.6	14.3	12.9	11.5	10.1
10.6	12.0	13.4	14.9	16.3	102	15.9	14.5	13.1	11.7	10.3
10.8	12.2	13.7	15.1	16.6	103	16.2	14.7	13.3	11.9	10.5
11.0	12.4	13.9	15.4	16.9	104	16.5	15.0	13.5	12.1	10.6
11.2	12.7	14.2	15.6	17.1	105	16.7	15.3	13.8	12.3	10.8
11.4	12.9	14.4	15.9	17.4	106	17.0	15.5	14.0	12.5	11.0
11.6	13.1	14.7	16.2	17.7	107	17.3	15.8	14.3	12.7	11.2
11.8	13.4	14.9	16.5	18.0	108	17.6	16.1	14.5	13.0	11.4
12.0	13.6	15.2	16.8	18.3	109	17.9	16.4	14.8	13.2	11.6
12.2	13.8	15.4	17.1	18.7	110	18.2	16.6	15.0	13.4	11.9

SD: standard deviation score (or Z-score). Although the interpretation of a fixed percent-of-median value varies across age and height, and generally the two scales cannot be compared, the approximate percent-of-median values for −1 and −2 SD are 90% and 80% of median, respectively (Gorstein J et al. Issues in the assessment of nutritional status using anthropometry. *Bulletin of the World Health Organization*, 1994, 72:273–283).

[a] Length is measured for children below 85 cm. For children 85 cm or more, height is measured. Recumbent length is on average 0.5 cm greater than standing height; although the difference is of no importance to individual children, a correction may be made by subtracting 0.5 cm from all lengths above 84.9 cm if standing height cannot be measured.

Appendix 2
Sample recording form

Sample recording form

Registration no.:	Unit no.:	Ward no.:
Patient's name:	Date of birth or age:	Sex: M/F
Mother's name:	Father's name:	Religion:
Next of kin (if different):	Relationship:	Head of household:

Address (including description of how to get to and recognize the house):

Date of admission:	Date of discharge:	Admitting doctor or nurse:

Cured: yes/no   Deceased: yes/no   Transferred: yes/no   Failed to return for follow-up: yes/no

Family information

Father's age:	Occupation:	
Mother's age:	Occupation:	No. of pregnancies:
No. of live births:	No. of living children:	Family planning: yes/no

If yes, specify: condoms/intra-uterine device/injectables/oral contraceptives/tubal ligation/other (specify)

Current carer of child: Educational level attained: primary/secondary/tertiary (university)

Reading ability: illiterate/poor/moderate/good

Monthly family income/support (in US$):

Land cultivated: yes/no   If yes, specify area cultivated (in m^2) and crops grown:

Type of housing: tent/hut/compound/house/other (specify)   No. of rooms:

No. of adults/children sharing housing:

Water supply: inside/outside/communal standpipe/well/spring   Distance from housing:

Sanitation facility: open defecation/shallow pit/pit latrine/pour–flush latrine/other (specify)

No. of families using sanitation facility:

Electricity supply: yes/no   If yes, specify electrical appliances: refrigerator/radio/television/other

Medical history

Complaints (list in order of importance)	Duration or age at which started

Describe current illness (circle whichever is appropriate):

Appetite: hungry/normal/poor/no appetite

Vomiting: yes/no

Diarrhoea: yes/no   Appearance: bloody/mucoid/watery/soft/solid/other (specify)

Intestinal parasites: yes/no

Oedema: none/feet/legs/face/abdomen/generalized   Intermittent: yes/no

Shortness of breath: yes/no   Cough: yes/no   Fever: yes/no

Skin changes: yes/no   If yes, describe:

Hair changes: yes/no   If yes, describe:

Weight loss: yes/no

Dietary history

Duration of exclusive breastfeeding (in months):

Total duration or age at which breastfeeding stopped:

Age at which non-milk feeds started:

Usual diet before current illness:

Type of food or fluid given	Age at which started (months)	Age at which stopped (months)	Amount per feed (g or ml)
Infant formula or animal milk (specify)			
Cereals (specify)			
Other staple foods[a] (specify)			
Water, herbal teas or other drinks (specify)			
Fresh fruit/fruit juice			
Orange and dark-green vegetables			
Other vegetables and pulses			
Fish, meat or eggs			
Other foods (specify)			

[a] Includes rice, corn, cassava, sorghum, potatoes and noodles.

Diet since current illness began (describe any changes):

Diet during past 24 hours (record all intake):

Immunization history

Immunization card: yes/no

Immunization	Date or age at which given[a]			
	First	Second	Third	Booster
BCG	At birth or >6 months	—	—	—
Polio	At birth	2 months	3 months	12 months
DTP	3 months	4 months	5 months	12 months
Measles	6 or 9 months	—	—	—

BCG: bacille Calmette–Guérin vaccine, DTP: diphtheria–tetanus–pertussis vaccine.
[a]Circle immunizations already given.

Physical examination

Date																				
Height (cm)																				
Weight^a (kg)																				
Weight-for-height (SD or %)																				
MUAC (cm)																				
MUAC-for-age (SD)																				
Oedema^b																				
Temperature (°C)																				

MUAC: mid-upper arm circumference.

^{a} These values should be recorded on a weight chart. A sample weight chart is given on page 49 (see also Fig. 1, page 22).

^{b} +++ = Severe oedema, ++ = moderate oedema, + = mild oedema.

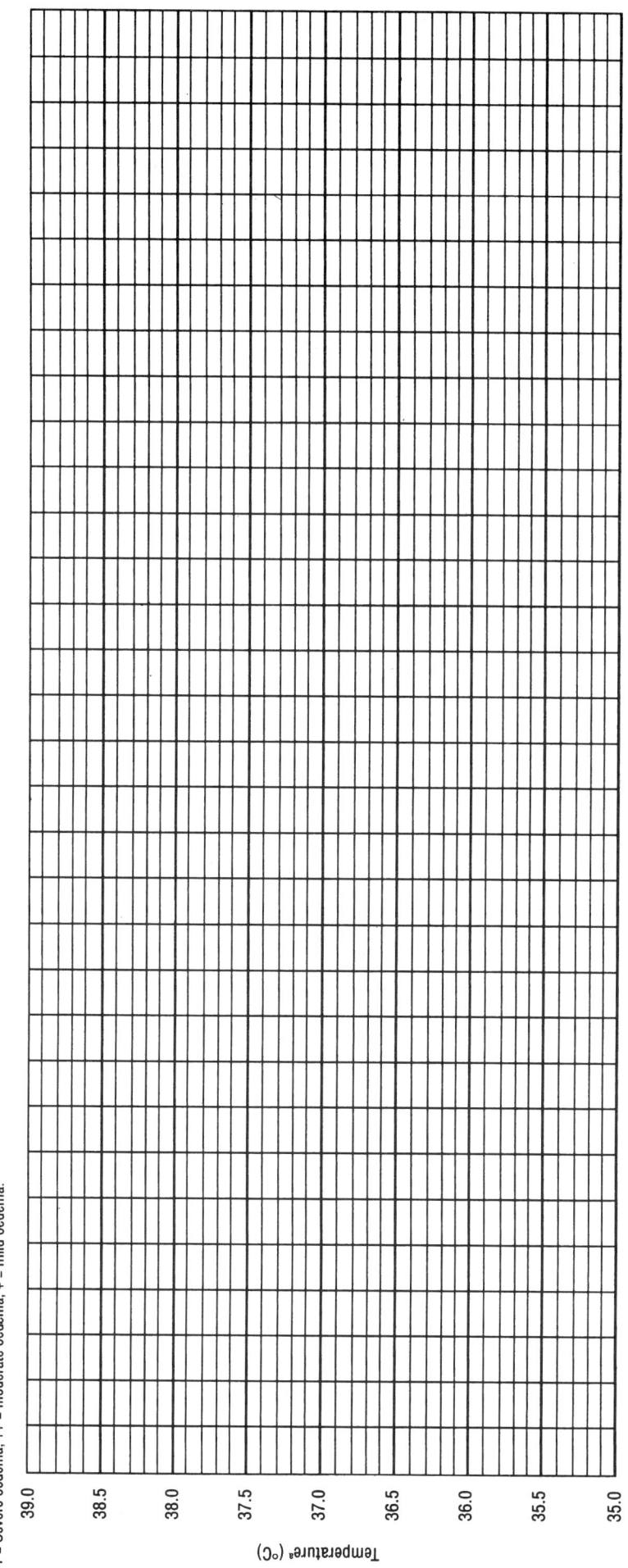

Temperature (°C): 39.0, 38.5, 38.0, 37.5, 37.0, 36.5, 36.0, 35.5, 35.0

^{a} The temperature should be taken at least twice daily (morning and afternoon). For each reading, the date and time (e.g. 31.8, 07:00h) and precise temperature should be plotted.

Diagnostic signs

Date																																
No. of stools/day																																
Dehydration[a]																																
No. of episodes of vomiting/day																																
Vol. of urine passed/day (ml)																																
Cough[a]																																
Anaemia[a]																																
Pulse rate (per min)																																
Respiratory rate (breaths/min)																																

Specific treatment[b]

[a] + = Sign present, — = sign absent.
[b] List any specific treatments given.

Sample food intake chart[a]

Date:

Feed: .... feeds of .... ml each = ... ml per day

Time	Type of feed	Amount offered (ml)	Amount left in cup (ml)	Amount taken by child (ml)	Estimated amount vomited (ml)	Watery diarrhoea (yes/no)
Total						

Total food intake over 24 hours (total amount taken − total amount vomited) = ... ml

[a] To be completed for each 24-hour period.

Appendix 2

Sample weight chart[a]

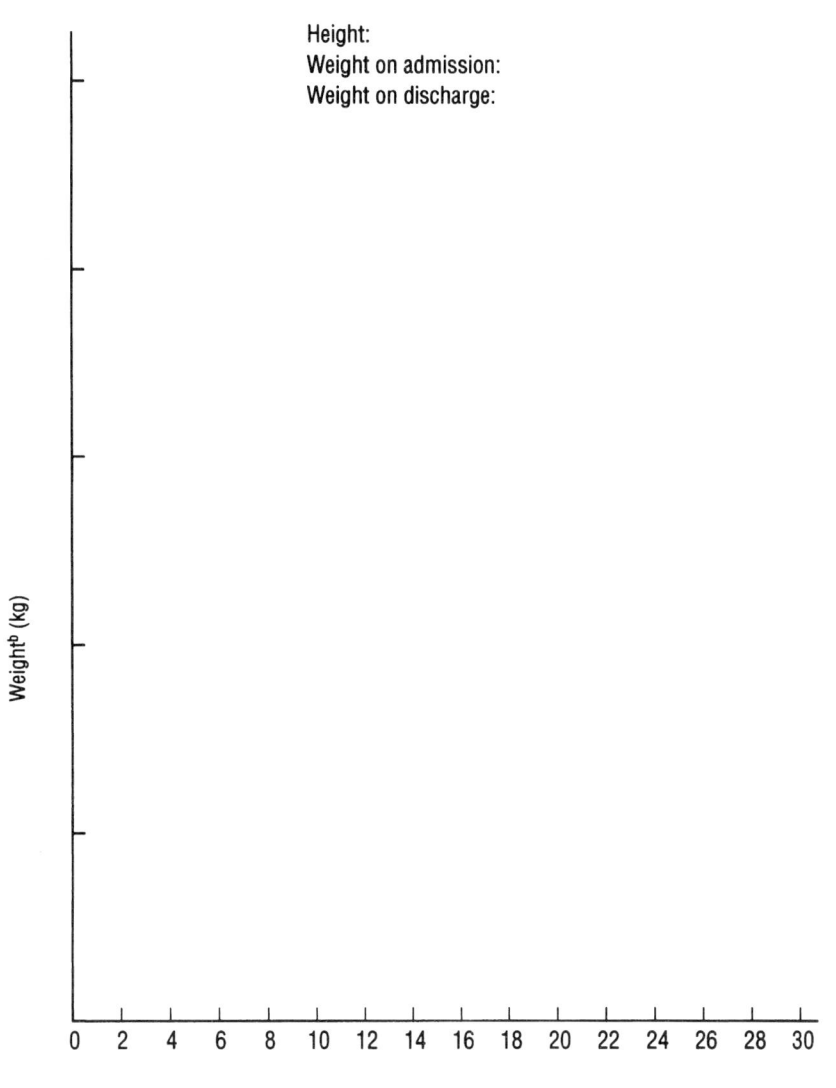

Height:
Weight on admission:
Weight on discharge:

Weight[b] (kg)

Time after admission (days)

[a] An example of a completed weight chart is given in Fig. 1 (page 22).

[b] Variable vertical axis. The divisions should be marked with the most appropriate scale.

Summary chart

	Date	Weight (kg)	Height (cm)	Oedema[a]	Height-for-age (SD or %)[b]	Weight-for-height (SD or %)[b]
Admission						
Discharge						
Follow-up						
Follow-up						
Follow-up						

[a] +++ = Severe oedema, ++ = moderate oedema, + = mild oedema.

[b] For further information, see Table 3 (page 4).

Observations

Appendix 3
Physiological basis for treatment of severe malnutrition

Affected organ or system	Effects	Treatment
Cardiovascular system	Cardiac output and stroke volume are reduced	If the child appears dehydrated, give ReSoMal or F-75 diet (see section 4.4 of the main text); do not give fluids intravenously unless the child is in shock
	Infusion of saline may cause an increase in venous pressure	
	Any increase in blood volume can easily produce acute heart failure; any decrease will further compromise tissue perfusion	Restrict blood transfusion to 10 ml/kg and give a diuretic
	Blood pressure is low	
	Renal perfusion and circulation time are reduced	
	Plasma volume is usually normal and red cell volume is reduced	
Liver	Synthesis of all proteins is reduced	Do not give the child large meals
	Abnormal metabolites of amino acids are produced	Ensure that the amount of protein given does not exceed the metabolic capacity of the liver, but is sufficient to support synthesis of proteins (1–2 g/kg per day)
	Capacity of liver to take up, metabolize and excrete toxins is severely reduced	
	Energy production from substrates such as galactose and fructose is much slower than normal	Reduce the dosage of drugs that depend on hepatic disposal or are hepatotoxic
	Gluconeogenesis is reduced, which increases the risk of hypoglycaemia during infection	Ensure that sufficient carbohydrate is given to avoid the need for gluconeogenesis
	Bile secretion is reduced	Do not give iron supplements, which may be dangerous because transferrin levels are reduced
Genitourinary system	Glomerular filtration is reduced	Prevent further tissue breakdown by treating any infections and providing adequate energy (80–100 kcal$_{th}$ or 336–420 kJ/kg per day)
	Capacity of kidney to excrete excess acid or a water load is greatly reduced	
	Urinary phosphate output is low	Do not give the child more protein than is required to maintain tissues
	Sodium excretion is reduced	
	Urinary tract infection is common	Ensure that high-quality proteins are given, with balanced amino acids
		Avoid nutrients that give an acid load, such as magnesium chloride

Affected organ or system	Effects	Treatment
Genitourinary system (*continued*)		Restrict dietary sodium (see Appendix 5)
		Ensure that water intake is sufficient but not excessive
Gastrointestinal system	Production of gastric acid is reduced	Give the child small, frequent feeds
	Intestinal motility is reduced	If absorption is poor, increase the frequency and reduce the size of each feed
	Pancreas is atrophied and production of digestive enzymes is reduced	
	Small intestinal mucosa is atrophied; secretion of digestive enzymes is reduced	If there is malabsorption of fat, treatment with pancreatic enzymes may be useful
	Absorption of nutrients is reduced when large amounts of food are eaten	
Immune system	All aspects of immunity are diminished	Treat all children with broad-spectrum antimicrobials (see Appendix 6 and section 4.6 of the main text)
	Lymph glands, tonsils and the thymus are atrophied	
	Cell-mediated (T-cell) immunity is severely depressed	Because of the risk of transmission of infection, ensure that newly admitted children are kept apart from children who are recovering from infection
	IgA levels in secretions are reduced	
	Complement components are low	
	Phagocytes do not kill ingested bacteria efficiently	
	Tissue damage does not result in inflammation or migration of white cells to the affected area	
	Acute phase immune response is diminished	
	Typical signs of infection, such as an increased white cell count and fever, are frequently absent	
	Hypoglycaemia and hypothermia are both signs of severe infection and are usually associated with septic shock	
Endocrine system	Insulin levels are reduced and the child has glucose intolerance	Give the child small, frequent feeds
		Do not give steroids
	Insulin growth factor 1 (IGF-1) levels are reduced, although growth hormone levels are increased	
	Cortisol levels are usually increased	
Circulatory system	Basic metabolic rate is reduced by about 30%	Keep the child warm to prevent hypothermia; dry the child quickly and properly after washing and cover with clothes and blankets, ensure that windows are kept closed at night and keep the temperature of the living environment at 25–30 °C
	Energy expenditure due to activity is very low	

Affected organ or system	Effects	Treatment
Circulatory system (*continued*)	Both heat generation and heat loss are impaired; the child becomes hypothermic in a cold environment and hyperthermic in a hot environment	If a child has fever, cool the child by sponging with tepid (not cold) water (*never* alcohol rubs)
Cellular function	Sodium pump activity is reduced and cell membranes are more permeable than normal, which leads to an increase in intracellular sodium and a decrease in intracellular potassium and magnesium Protein synthesis is reduced	Give large doses of potassium and magnesium to all children (see Appendix 5) Restrict sodium intake (see Appendix 5)
Skin, muscles and glands	The skin and subcutaneous fat are atrophied, which leads to loose folds of skin Many signs of dehydration are unreliable; eyes may be sunken because of loss of subcutaneous fat in the orbit Many glands, including the sweat, tear and salivary glands, are atrophied; the child has dryness of the mouth and eyes and sweat production is reduced Respiratory muscles are easily fatigued; the child is lacking in energy	Rehydrate the child with ReSoMal or F-75 diet (see section 4.4 of the main text)

Appendix 4
Composition of mineral and vitamin mixes

Composition of mineral mix solution

Substance	Amount
Potassium chloride	89.5 g
Tripotassium citrate	32.4 g
Magnesium chloride ($MgCl_2 \cdot 6H_2O$)	30.5 g
Zinc acetate	3.3 g
Copper sulfate	0.56 g
Sodium selenate[a]	10 mg
Potassium iodide[a]	5 mg
Water to make	1000 ml

[a] If it is not possible to weigh very small amounts accurately, this substance may be omitted.

The above solution can be stored at room temperature. It is added to ReSoMal or liquid feed at a concentration of 20 ml/litre.

Composition of vitamin mix

Vitamin	Amount per litre of liquid diet
Water-soluble:	
Thiamine (vitamin B_1)	0.7 mg
Riboflavin (vitamin B_2)	2.0 mg
Nicotinic acid	10 mg
Pyridoxine (vitamin B_6)	0.7 mg
Cyanocobalamin (vitamin B_{12})	1 µg
Folic acid	0.35 mg
Ascorbic acid (vitamin C)	100 mg
Pantothenic acid (vitamin B_5)	3 mg
Biotin	0.1 mg
Fat-soluble:	
Retinol (vitamin A)	1.5 mg
Calciferol (vitamin D)	30 µg
α-Tocopherol (vitamin E)	22 mg
Vitamin K	40 µg

Appendix 5

Desirable daily nutrient intake during initial phase of treatment

Nutrient	Amount per kg of body weight
Water	120–140 ml
Energy	100 kcal$_{th}$ (420 kJ)
Protein	1–2 g
Electrolytes:	
Sodium	1.0 mmol (23 mg)[a]
Potassium	4.0 mmol (160 mg)
Magnesium	0.6 mmol (10 mg)
Phosphorus	2.0 mmol (60 mg)
Calcium	2.0 mmol (80 mg)
Trace minerals:	
Zinc	30 µmol (2.0 mg)
Copper	4.5 µmol (0.3 mg)
Selenium	60 nmol (4.7 µg)
Iodine	0.1 µmol (12 µg)
Water-soluble vitamins:	
Thiamine (vitamin B$_1$)	70 µg
Riboflavin (vitamin B$_2$)	0.2 mg
Nicotinic acid	1 mg
Pyridoxine (vitamin B$_6$)	70 µg
Cyanocobalamin (vitamin B$_{12}$)	0.1 mg
Folic acid	0.1 mg
Ascorbic acid (vitamin C)	10 µg
Pantothenic acid (vitamin B$_5$)	0.3 mg
Biotin	10 µg
Fat-soluble vitamins:	
Retinol (vitamin A)	0.15 mg
Calciferol (vitamin D)	3 µg
α-Tocopherol (vitamin E)	2.2 mg
Vitamin K	4 µg

[a] Value refers to the *maximum* recommended daily intake.

Appendix 6
Drug dosages for treatment of infections

Drugs for treatment of infections in severely malnourished children[a,b]

Antimicrobial	Dosage	Dosage form
Amoxicillin	15 mg/kg orally every 8 hours	tablet, 250 mg (anhydrous) syrup, 250 mg/5 ml
Ampicillin	25 mg/kg orally every 6 hours[c] 50 mg/kg IM or IV every 6 hours	tablet, 250 mg powder for injection, 500 mg (as sodium salt) in vial, mixed with 2.5 ml of sterile water
Benzylpenicillin	50 000 IU/kg IM or IV every 6 hours	powder for injection, 600 mg (= 1 million IU) (as sodium or potassium salt), mixed with 1.6 ml of sterile water (for IM injection) or 10 ml of sterile water (for IV injection)
Chloramphenicol	25 mg/kg IM or IV every 6 hours (for meningitis only) or every 8 hours (for other conditions)	powder for injection, 1 g (as sodium succinate) in vial, mixed with 3.2 ml of sterile water (for IM injection) or 9.2 ml of sterile water (for IV injection)
Cotrimoxazole	25 mg of sulfamethoxazole + 5 mg of trimethoprim/kg orally every 12 hours	paediatric tablet, 100 mg of sulfamethoxazole + 20 mg of trimethoprim syrup, 200 mg of sulfamethoxazole + 40 mg of trimethoprim/5 ml
Gentamicin	7.5 mg/kg IM or IV once daily	injection, 10 mg (as sulfate)/ml in 1-ml vial injection, 20 mg, 40 mg, 80 mg (as sulfate)/ml in 2-ml vial
Metronidazole	Amoebiasis: 10 mg/kg orally every 8 hours for 5–10 days Giardiasis: 5 mg/kg orally every 8 hours for 5 days	tablet, 200 mg, 400 mg
Nalidixic acid	15 mg/kg orally every 6 hours	tablet, 250 mg

IM: intramuscularly, IV: intravenously.
[a] The drug dosages should be calculated on the basis of the child's weight, *never* the child's age.
[b] For further information see sections 4.6 and 7.3.
[c] Some institutions routinely give malnourished children higher doses of oral ampicillin (e.g. 50 mg/kg every 6 hours) because of poor absorption, although there is no evidence that these doses are more effective.

Drugs for treatment of tuberculosis in severely malnourished children[a]

Drug	Mode of action	Recommended dose (mg/kg)		
		Daily	Three times weekly	Twice weekly[b]
Isoniazid	bactericidal	5	10	15
Rifampicin	bactericidal	10	10	10
Pyrazinamide	bactericidal	25	35	50
Ethambutol	bacteriostatic	15	30	45

[a] For further information, see reference *1*.
[b] WHO does not generally recommend twice weekly regimens. If a patient receiving treatment twice weekly misses a dose, the missed dose represents a larger fraction of the total number of treatment doses than if the patient were receiving treatment three times weekly or daily. There is therefore a greater risk of treatment failure.

Drugs for treatment of helminthiasis in severely malnourished children[a]

Drug	Dosage	Specific indications
Albendazole	Children over 2 years: 400 mg in a single dose	Ascariasis, hookworm infections, trichuriasis and strongyloidiasis
Ivermectin	200 µg/kg in a single dose	Strongyloidiasis
Levamisole	2.5 mg/kg in a single dose	Ascariasis, hookworm infections and trichuriasis
Mebendazole	Children over 2 years: 100 mg twice daily for 3 days for inpatient treatment or 500 mg in a single dose for outpatient treatment	Ascariasis, hookworm infections and trichuriasis
Piperazine	Children aged 2–12 years: 75 mg/kg in a single dose to a maximum of 2.5 g	Ascariasis and trichuriasis
	Children under 2 years: 50 mg/kg in a single dose administered under medical supervision	
Pyrantel	10 mg/kg in a single dose	Ascariasis and hookworm infections

[a] For further information, see pages 32–33 and reference 2.

Drugs for treatment of malaria in severely malnourished children[a]

Drug	Dosage
Plasmodium malariae, P. ovale and susceptible forms of P. vivax malaria:	
Chloroquine	Total dose: 25 mg of base/kg orally given over 3 days Days 1 and 2: 10 mg of base/kg in a single dose Day 3: 5 mg of base/kg in a single dose
P. falciparum malaria:[b]	
Chloroquine	Total dose: 25 mg of base/kg orally given over 3 days Days 1 and 2: 10 mg of base/kg in a single dose Day 3: 5 mg of base/kg in a single dose
Quinine	8 mg of base/kg orally every 8 hours for 7 days
Pyrimethamine + sulfadoxine	Children: 5–10 kg: 12.5 mg + 250 mg orally in a single dose 11–20 kg: 25 mg + 500 mg orally in a single dose

[a] For further information, see page 33 and reference 3.
[b] The choice of drug should be based on national recommendations.

References

1. *Treatment of tuberculosis: guidelines for national programmes*, 2nd ed. Geneva, World Health Organization, 1997 (unpublished document WHO/TB/97.220; available on request from Global Tuberculosis Programme, World Health Organization, 1211 Geneva 27, Switzerland).

2. *Report of the WHO informal consultation on the use of chemotherapy for the control of morbidity due to soil-transmitted nematodes in humans, Geneva, 29 April to 1 May 1996.* Geneva, World Health Organization, 1996 (unpublished document WHO/CTD/SIP/96.2; available on request from Division of Control of Tropical Diseases, World Health Organization, 1211 Geneva 27, Switzerland).

Appendix 6

3. *Management of uncomplicated malaria and the use of antimalarial drugs for the protection of travellers. Report of an informal consultation, Geneva, 18–21 September 1995.* Geneva, World Health Organization, 1996 (unpublished document WHO/MAL/96.1075 Rev. 1; available on request from Division of Control of Tropical Diseases, World Health Organization, 1211 Geneva 27, Switzerland).

Appendix 7
Toys for severely malnourished children

Ring on a string (from 6 months)
Thread cotton reels and other small objects (e.g. cut from the neck of plastic bottles) on to a string. Tie the string in a ring, leaving a long piece of string hanging.

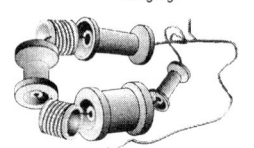

Rattle (from 12 months)
Cut long strips of plastic from coloured plastic bottles. Place them in a small transparent plastic bottle and glue the top on firmly.

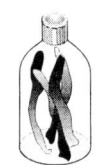

Drum (from 12 months)
Any tin with a tightly fitting lid.

Mirror (from 18 months)
A tin lid with no sharp edges.

In-and-out toy (from 9 months)
Any plastic or cardboard container and small objects (not small enough to be swallowed).

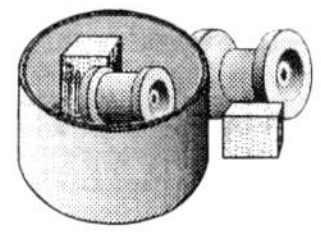

Posting bottle (from 12 months)
A large transparent plastic bottle with a small neck and small long objects that fit through the neck (not small enough to be swallowed).

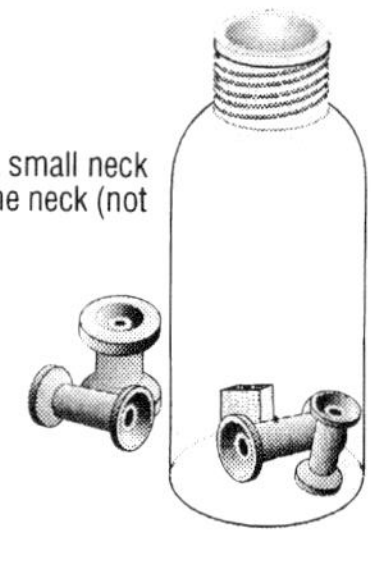

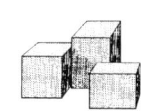

Blocks (from 9 months)
Small blocks of wood. Smooth the surfaces with sandpaper and paint in bright colours, if possible.

Push-along toy (from 12 months)
Make a hole in the centre of the base and lid of a cylindrical-shaped tin. Thread a piece of wire (about 60 cm long) through each hole and tie the ends inside the tin. Put some metal bottle tops inside the tin and close the lid.

Stacking bottle tops (from 12 months)
Cut at least three identical round plastic bottles in half and stack them.

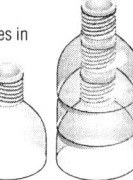

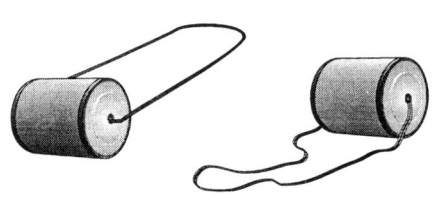

Pull-along toy (from 12 months)
As above, except that string is used instead of wire.

Nesting toys (from 9 months)
Cut off the bottom of two bottles of identical shape, but different size. The smaller bottle should be placed inside the larger bottle.

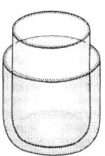

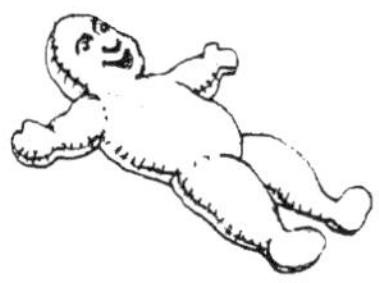

Puzzle (from 18 months)
Draw a figure (e.g. a doll) in a crayon on a square- or rectangular-shaped piece of cardboard. Cut the figure in half or quarters.

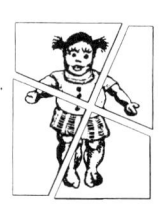

Doll (from 12 months)
Cut out two doll shapes from a piece of cloth and sew the edges together, leaving a small opening. Turn the doll inside-out and stuff with scraps of materials. Stitch up the opening and sew or draw a face on the doll.

Book (from 18 months)
Cut out three rectangular-shaped pieces of the same size from a cardboard box. Glue or draw a picture on both sides of each piece. Make two holes down one side of each piece and thread string through to make a book.

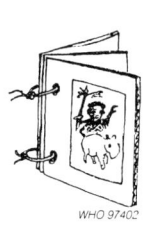

Appendix 8
Sample curriculum for play therapy

Each play session should include language and motor activities, and activities with toys. Teach the games or skills listed below when the child is ready for them. Encourage the child to use appropriate words to describe what he or she is doing.

Language activities (from 12 months)

At every play session, teach the child local songs, and games using the fingers and toes. Encourage the child to laugh, vocalize and describe what he or she is doing. Teach the child to use words such as *bang* when beating the drum, *bye* when waving goodbye, and *thank you* when given something.

Motor activities (from 6 months)

Always encourage the child to perform the next appropriate motor activity. For example, bounce the child up and down and hold the child under the arms so the child's feet support his or her weight. Help the child to sit up by propping him or her up with cushions or any other appropriate materials. Roll toys out of reach to encourage the child to crawl after them. Hold the child's hands and help him or her to walk. As soon as the child has started to walk unaided, give the child a push-along toy and later a pull-along toy (see Appendix 7).

Activities with toys[1]

Ring on a string (from 6 months)

1. Swing a ring on a string within reach of the child and encourage him or her to reach for it.
2. Suspend the ring over the crib and encourage the child to knock it and make it swing.
3. Let the child examine the ring. Then place the ring a short distance from the child, leaving the string within reach of the child. Teach the child to get the ring by pulling on the string.
4. Sit the child on your lap. Then, holding the string, lower the ring towards the floor. Teach the child to get the ring by pulling on the string. Also teach the child to dangle the ring.

Rattle and drum (from 12 months)

1. Let the child examine the rattle. Teach the child to use the word *shake* when shaking the rattle.
2. Encourage the child to beat the drum with the rattle. Teach the child to use the word *bang* when beating the drum.
3. Roll the drum out of the child's reach and encourage him or her to crawl after it.

---
[1] See Appendix 7.

In-and-out toy with blocks (from 9 months)

1. Let the child examine the container and blocks. Put the blocks into the container and shake it. Then teach the child to take them out, one at a time. Teach the child the meaning of the words *out* and *give*.
2. Teach the child to take out the blocks by turning the container upside-down.
3. Teach the child to hold a block in each hand and to bang the blocks together.
4. Teach the child to put the blocks in the container and to take them out again. Teach the child to use the words *in* and *out*.
5. Cover the blocks with the container and let the child find them. Then hide them under two or three covers or pieces of cloth and repeat the game. Teach the child to use the word *under*.
6. Turn the container upside-down and teach the child to put blocks on top of it.
7. Teach the child to stack the blocks, first two, then gradually more. Teach the child to use the words *up* when stacking the blocks and *down* when knocking them down.
8. Line up the blocks horizontally, first two, then more. Teach the child to push them along, making train or car noises. For children aged 18 months or more, teach the meaning of the words *stop, go, fast, slow* and *next to*. Then teach the child to sort the blocks by colours, first two colours, then more. Teach the meaning of the words *high* and *low*. Make up games.

Posting bottle (from 12 months)

Put some objects into a bottle. Shake it. Teach the child to turn the bottle upside-down and empty out the objects. Then teach the child to put the objects into the bottle and to take them out again. Try the same game again with different objects.

Stacking bottle tops (from 12 months)

Let the child play with two bottle tops. Then teach the child to stack them. Later increase the number of bottle tops. Teach children over 18 months to sort the bottle tops by colour and to use the words *high* and *low* when describing the stacks.

Doll (from 12 months)

Encourage the child to hold the doll. Teach the child to identify his or her own body parts and those of the doll when you name them. Teach children over 2 years to name their own body parts. Put the doll in a box for a bed and teach the child the words *bed* and *sleep*.

Books (from 18 months)

Sit the child on your lap. Teach the child to turn the pages of the book and to point to the pictures. Then teach the child to point to the pictures that you name. Talk about the pictures. Show the child pictures of simple familiar objects and of people and animals. Teach children over 2 years to name the pictures and to talk about them.